MORRIS AUTOMATED INFORMATION NETWORK

0 1029 0565721 3

T3-BNM-906

449 HALSEY ROAD
PARSIPPANY, NJ 07054
973-887-5150

JAN 0 5 2010   WITHDRAWN

eye of the beholder

TRUE STORIES OF PEOPLE
WITH FACIAL DIFFERENCES

laura greenwald

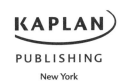

KAPLAN

PUBLISHING

New York

This publication is designed to provide accurate and authoritative information in regard to the subject matter covered. It is sold with the understanding that the publisher is not engaged in rendering legal, accounting, or other professional service. If legal advice or other expert assistance is required, the services of a competent professional should be sought.

© 2009 Laura Greenwald

Published by Kaplan Publishing, a division of Kaplan, Inc.
1 Liberty Plaza, 24th Floor
New York, NY 10006

All rights reserved. The text of this publication, or any part thereof, may not be reproduced in any manner whatsoever without written permission from the publisher.

Library of Congress Cataloging-in-Publication Data

Greenwald, Laura, 1963-
  Eye of the beholder : true stories of people with facial differences / Laura Greenwald.
    p. cm.
  Includes bibliographical references.
  ISBN 978-1-60714-083-2
  1. Face--Abnormalities--Patients--Biography. 2. Face--Wounds and injuries--Patients--Biography. I. Title.
  QM695.F32G74 2009
  617.5'20440922--dc22
  [B]
                                    2009007256

Printed in the United States of America

10 9 8 7 6 5 4 3 2 1

ISBN: 978-1-60714-083-2

Kaplan Publishing books are available at special quantity discounts to use for sales promotions, employee premiums, or educational purposes. Please e-mail our Special Sales Department to order or for more information at kaplanpublishing@kaplan.com, or write to Kaplan Publishing, 1 Liberty Plaza, 24th Floor, New York, NY 10006.

God made man because he loves stories.

—Elie Wiesel, "The Gates of the Forest"

⚬

A portion of the author's proceeds benefits programs
to support people with facial differences.

⚬

CONTENTS

FOREWORD

In *Eye of the Beholder*, Laura Greenwald captures the spirit and voices of people with facial differences and their families, and gives us insight into the many issues they face in their everyday journeys. The "difference" that distinguishes each of these people is a facial anomaly: a facial difference acquired through birth, illness, or accident.

My interest in facial differences began in 1992, when I joined the board of Forward Face. Forward Face is a nonprofit organization in New York City that provides children and their families support to manage the medical and social effects of facial differences. The organization provides educational materials and networking for parents, raises public awareness, and sponsors Inner Faces, a support group for teens and adults with facial differences.

I volunteered to facilitate a series of communication and social skills workshops for the Inner Faces. Much time at the workshops was spent designing and performing role-plays. I was surprised at how much the Inner Faces enjoyed role-playing and how good they were at it. One of the members of the group suggested we enhance some of the role-plays to illustrate what the group had learned and perform them in front of an audience.

Early in my studies at the Fielding Graduate Institute, I was introduced to the work of Auguste Boal and the transformative power of the Theatre of the Oppressed. The convergence of my attendance at the Boal workshop and the group's interest in performing planted the seed that grew into a full-blown theater project, based on Boal's work. The

Inner Faces made a commitment to do participatory theater: to write, produce, and act in an original musical presentation, based on the stories of their lives growing up with facial differences.

The members of the Inner Faces began to believe in their ability to relate in the world and started to take a variety of risks. They were transformed and motivated by their theater work to help themselves, as well as to help others. With anticipation, fear, and much excitement, the Inner Faces performed their original musical, *Let's Face the Music*, to a packed audience on an off-Broadway stage in Tribeca. They received a standing ovation at every performance and much praise and recognition for their courage and accomplishment from strangers, friends, and family. Their stories and their voices were heard.

The next step was education to bring about social change and improve the quality of life for people with facial differences. The Inner Faces inspired me to write my dissertation about our theater project and transformation.

We developed the documentary *Face, a Portrait*, which is the centerpiece of "Appreciating Differences," our educational program targeted to middle and high school students. The documentary has been aired on public television both nationally and internationally and is being shown in more than 4,000 schools all over the country.

A few years later, the Inner Faces performed their second participatory theater project, *Phoenix Café*, in an off-Broadway theater on Manhattan's Upper West Side. Eight new members joined seven of the original cast. Since then, several of the members have developed into staunch social advocates and continually participate in programs in schools and universities, educating others about difference.

The members of the Inner Faces presently are involved in writing and producing an educational video for medical students who are interested in reconstructive surgery. The students will hear an honest and open discussion based on the real experiences of craniofacial patients. The Inner Faces will discuss what is important and often overlooked in the patient–doctor relationship. We will travel to many medical schools, show the video, and engage in an open dialogue with the medical community.

I have mentored and advised the Inner Faces for the last 14 years. Our legacy of caring, humanity, and love is being passed on through the group's evolving leadership.

In *Eye of the Beholder*, Laura Greenwald offers us the opportunity to learn more about facial differences by journeying with several people as they courageously search for acceptance and a life of dignity. In her timely book, Laura illustrates many of the issues surrounding facial differences: the different kinds of family support needed; the trauma of surgeries; the day-to-day contact with harassment and staring; the isolation and silence; and the difficulties in dealing with communication, relationships, and employment. She addresses the latest medical information from experts involved in all aspects of the field.

Eye of the Beholder helps people with facial differences move out of the shadows and into the spotlight. We are privileged to hear their voices. Laura is a compassionate and elegant writer who pays attention to the voices of these people and offers them center stage. I am thrilled that finally there is a comprehensive book that educates us on the many issues concerning facial differences and allows us to hear voices that might otherwise have been silent. Professionals and laypersons alike will learn and be inspired by this scholarly and heartfelt presentation.

Jodie Berlin Morrow, PhD
New York City

Look at me and really see
The kindness in my eyes,
The smile that twitches at my mouth —
The fear that makes me shy.

Look at me and disregard
Those differences that stand,
Invisible as winter winds
And strong as steel bands.

When you look at me is all you find
The measure of my face?
Against some standard I can't meet —
Do I lose the human race?

Do you see the things that I can't change?
Do you gaze and look away?
It's lonely here without your eyes.
One look — then turn away?

The beauty of the human soul
Is not the pretty face.
It's found within the heart and hands
Of those who look — and stay.

— Jeff Moyer, son of Jack Moyer
(Chapter 7), January 2005

The perfect human being is uninteresting.

— Joseph Campbell

INTRODUCTION

HAVE YOU EVER RUN into someone whose face looked markedly different from those of others? Perhaps it was a child with something as common as a cleft lip. You stared for a few seconds and then turned away. Perhaps it was someone whose face was badly scarred from a fire. Maybe you couldn't stop staring. Either way, you probably felt uneasy and avoided any interaction with that person. Why? Because you didn't know what to say? Because you felt that somehow you would have to acknowledge the difference? Would you have the same reaction to a person in a wheelchair or a person missing an arm?

Even with all their variations, we know that faces are supposed to look a certain way. When we see one that doesn't fit our image of "usual," we're tripped up. For any object, whether it's a spoon or a car or a face, we're given visual clues so we can identify it easily. These visual clues help us to form an archetype of the image, a frame of reference. Once we know the archetype of a spoon, for example — a long handle attached to a shallow bowl, usually made of metal — we can easily identify all types of spoons, from simple to ornate to downright funky. When confronted with a spoon that is unlike its archetype and unlike all others we've seen, it's likely we would spend some time observing it. It's the same with cars; it's the same with faces.

In his best-selling book *Blink*, Malcolm Gladwell writes, "If you were to approach a one-year-old child who sits playing on the floor and do something a little bit puzzling, such as cupping your hands over hers, the child would immediately look up into your eyes. Why? Because what you have done requires explanation, and the child knows that she can find an answer on your face."

The face is our center of communication. Four of the five senses are located on the face, and behind it is the brain, where all stimuli are processed. (If our eyes were in our bellies, then our midriffs would be the focal point, and this book might be about abdominal scars, belly rings, and stretch marks.) A facial difference interrupts the communication flow. Depending on the extent of the disfigurement, the interruption may be like a flickering light during a storm, or it might be a blackout.

Unlike other disfigurements, a facial difference is more than a temporary distraction because the face is the focal point of every person, the first part with which we make a connection. How faces appear to others provides context, giving others a starting point for forming assumptions, judgments, and beliefs.

When people meet, shake hands, and look into each other's eyes, they anticipate seeing an archetypal face. When that expectation isn't met, their brains need a moment to adjust. For someone who is facially different, every social encounter is a risk, a dare, with an unknown outcome.

Nichola Rumsey, PhD, co-editor of *Visibly Different: Coping with Disfigurement*, found that in social situations, people stand a foot farther away from people who are disfigured. "If you take a good step backward, it changes the feeling between the two people, so it's less personal and more distant," she wrote.

Andi (not her real name) was teased mercilessly while growing up, especially at school and at summer camp. Born with a cleft lip and a small left eye, from which she cannot see, Andi, now in her early forties, thinks that in many ways the teasing wasn't done with the intent to harm. Other children just didn't know how to understand and respond to her facial difference.

"A lot of teasing comes from one's fear of the unknown and ignorance," she says, adding that if other people don't know what's wrong with you, you become a target.

At summer camp, the other kids would harass her, whisper about her, or just plain ignore her. Most of the torture, as Andi calls it, happened when the camp counselors weren't around. When the counselors were present, the children behaved in a civil manner toward Andi. Consequently, when she complained, the counselors didn't believe her. At one point, her parents came to camp to see what was going on; the children couldn't have been more well-behaved and mannerly.

"I started to think, is it me?" she says. "Maybe if I do something different, it will get better." She's not sure whether it did or not, because she's spent a lot of energy trying to block out those memories.

Teasing may not seem so harmful. After all, people tease each other all the time, just out of playfulness. But when teasing is constant, meanspirited, and results in alienation, it causes deep psychological wounds that can stay with a person forever. Andi coped by developing a thick skin. She created a wall around herself to shut others out, essentially alienating herself on what felt like her own terms. She was left feeling lonely, unwanted, and unworthy.

She also suppressed all her emotions, even learning not to cry. As an adolescent, she traded tears for panic attacks and coughing jags when she felt upset. Decades later, Andi still has a difficult time showing her emotions. She struggles to cry at appropriate times, such as during sad movies, funerals, or weddings. She has trouble connecting with others, and having physical contact with someone is almost out of the question. Even exchanging a hug with a good friend feels risky. Andi knows her behavior is unhealthy, but she cannot escape the susurrations, the whispers that follow her everywhere, telling her she's different.

Rather than focus on what she cannot yet do, Andi is working to raise public awareness and to alleviate the stigma that people with facial differences encounter. She participated in a video project that has been distributed for free to more than 2,500 schools across the United States. She visits schools in her hometown and leads dialogues about the video and about people with facial differences. Everyone can somehow relate to the video because everyone has insecurities. "It's amazing every time. That's what's so powerful," she says. "The themes are universal."

She tries to educate parents to address difficult issues such as facial differences. When children ask questions about someone who looks different from them, the typical parental response is to hush them up. Parents say, "Don't stare; don't ask." Andi explains: "They shush them up, and then it's a scary thing."

When Andi's niece was young, Andi made a special effort to educate her about facial difference. She started by showing her niece the hearing aid she wears. "Now, it's no big deal. When you make something no big deal, it becomes no big deal," she says.

Andi also helped create a special curriculum for elementary school children, with the hope that by being educated about differences early, they will be less likely to tease others and will learn to come to the defense of children who are targets. "Education and awareness conquer ignorance," she says. "I would never want another child to go through what I did. I can't make it go away, but I can make a difference."

Facial differences give us pause because they are a reminder that things can go wrong, making us feel vulnerable. Babies are born disfigured from no less than two dozen craniofacial syndromes; the more commonly known include Apert syndrome, cleft lip and palate, craniosynostosis, and hydrocephalus. Tragic accidents also occur and serious diseases strike. The world is chaotic and full of uncertainty.

It's difficult to say how many people are affected by a facial difference. In 2006, the U.S. Centers for Disease Control released statistics on birth defects for the country. Birth defects of the face and mouth are the most common. Each year, more than 6,700 babies are born with cleft lip, cleft palate, or both. Fewer than 1,000 babies every year are born with some type of eye defect. Some states don't track birth defects, so the CDC relies on data from 11 states (Alabama, Arkansas, California, Georgia, Hawaii, Iowa, Massachusetts, North Carolina, Oklahoma, Texas, and Utah) to come up with its national estimates.

Advances in medicine and science have helped a great number of people with facial differences achieve a quality of life that would have been impossible even several years ago, but everything has limitations. For some, the financial cost is too high; for others, the necessary resources aren't readily available. For too many, a medical "fix" simply is not possible. Still others have accepted their difference or, after many attempts at a correction, have reached a saturation point. Sometimes it's enough that function is restored; form takes a backseat or never even climbs aboard.

Even though all of us have imperfections, some physical and some not, most of us can hide them. A missing leg may be covered by pants, and a bad liver is tucked safely inside the gut. A disobedient temper may strike only behind a closed door. Most of the time, we can pretend our imperfections don't exist, or we can at least feel safe knowing they're well hidden. We have the luxury of bringing them out if and when we choose. ("Did I tell you about my bad heart?") Not so with facial differences. They're exposed for all to see. So imagine that we had to wear our imperfections like labels on our faces every day, all the time — in photos, at formal events, interviewing for a job, and meeting someone for the first time. What if we had no way to hide our imperfections? We would struggle with feeling self-conscious, and we would constantly wonder how we were being judged by others.

My husband is a down-to-earth, gregarious type who warms up to people quickly and talks to strangers regularly. During the time I was writing this book, he had oral surgery, leaving his face swollen and bruised for several days. Though it was a temporary situation, he felt self-conscious about it and made a discovery that startled him. Subconsciously, he stopped making small talk with strangers, and he even avoided making eye contact with people — in effect, alienating himself.

This because of some temporary bruising and swelling! No one who saw him ran away in horror, yet he felt an odd duty to protect others from seeing him, as though he would be responsible for their disgust if they did.

In a very real sense, our faces are our identities and when we suffer an insult to the face, it feels more personal than an injury to most other parts of our body. An injury to the arm or foot, for example, is an injury to a body part, but an injury to the face is a violation of self. People who acquire a facial difference through an accident or disease must come to terms with seeing a new self in the mirror every day. Their new face may not reflect their emotions the same way their old face did — a 100-watt smile is now a crooked frown — and they may struggle to fit into their new self.

Some people with facial differences also have impaired senses, giving them an added level of disconnectedness. For example, children with cleft lip and palate often are hearing-impaired, making it much harder to engage in conversation with hearing people. Some people who have suffered trauma to their mouths and jaws lose their sense of smell or taste and may have a hard time speaking, another barrier to communication. Those with severe eye injuries often have impaired vision or no vision. Not only are those with facial differences alienated because of their appearance, but if they're also sensory-impaired, they're pushed even farther from the circle of humanity.

David Roche is disfigured. He was born with a large benign tumor on the left side of his face and neck. Attempts at treatment when he was an infant left his face permanently damaged. He took his disability public, becoming a speaker, humorist, performer, and teacher. "To survive spiritually and emotionally, I have been forced to find my own inner beauty. I have discovered that I am a child of God. I am whole," he says. "And my face is a gift."

David, whose keen eyes reflect a kind of sacred humanness, uses his gift to lift others, even those without facial differences who are lucky enough to hear him speak. At 64, he's grown to understand that his feelings are universal. Being facially different makes him more credible, but everyone has a fear of being unworthy, of not being good enough, or of being abandoned. Hold up a mirror to someone who feels vulnerable because she's too tall, too short, too fat, too skinny, or not pretty enough and you'll see your own reflection. We have a kind of Goldilocks syndrome: We're never just right. All of us, at one time or another, have felt vulnerable, not good enough, a misfit in our own skin. We've felt insignificant, worthless. That, says David, is the real disfigurement.

Why measure ourselves against others or against society's ideals? Does it help us to become better people, or does it drive us to become neurotic, self-absorbed, and shallow? Is perfection — assuming it is attainable — a worthy goal? Is there a reason that we're all different, imperfect in so many ways? Still, imagine if you're behind the curve. Unlike the young athlete who isn't fully satisfied with the development of his calves or the middle-aged woman who is discouraged by her sagging breasts, people with facial differences must face the very real effects of how others perceive and treat them. Most people with a facial difference will say, "If you can't accept me, that's your problem, not mine." But that's not entirely true. Treating someone poorly can leave a lasting mark. But before we beat ourselves up too much, perhaps it's because we struggle to accept ourselves that we stumble when we try to accept others.

The desire to fit in is powerful. Repeatedly hitting social barriers begins to feel like banishment, which is a harsh punishment typically reserved for evildoers. Shakespeare's Romeo, who was banished from Verona because of his love for Juliet, cried desperately that "the damned use that word in hell." Banishment may be an appropriate penalty for convicted criminals, but not for lovers or for people with physical differences.

In this book, you'll find stories of people who have varying degrees of disfigurement. Many were born with their differences, so they've grown up with the only face they've ever known. Some acquired a difference through disease or trauma, and their focus shifted between a desire to look the way they had and a desire to survive. This group in particular experiences a unique psychology.

In May 2005, researchers from the Yale School of Medicine reported that "patients disfigured in traumatic incidents are much more likely to suffer post-traumatic stress disorder, unemployment, marital problems, binge drinking, and depression." People born with a difference don't know anything else, and they have a head start learning how to cope, whereas people who become disfigured as a result of a traumatic accident must cope not only with the injury but also with the desire to be how they once were. With an acquired difference, there is a greater expectation that the injuries and their aftermath might be completely repaired, until eventually the reality of "good enough" settles in and they take what they've gained and move forward.

The people highlighted in this book were called on a journey. None of them asked to go. And despite their individual outcomes, all of them found more of themselves on their journey than they had originally lost. They accepted the challenge of the journey and, as a result, discovered the power of inner beauty, the healing that accompanies acceptance, and the value of courage in the face of rejection. Their stories lift us and show us what it's like to be extraordinary.

⌘

CHAPTER 1

nothing is normal

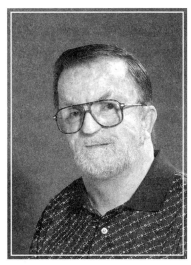

Bill Costa

We restore, repair, and make whole those parts…
which nature has given but fortune has taken away,
not so much that they may delight the eye but that they may buoy up
the spirit and help the mind of the afflicted.

—Gaspare Tagliacozzi (1597)

BILL COSTA RECALLS the first thing that popped into his mind when his dermatologist told him he would probably lose his entire nose. It had nothing to do with how he might look, how much pain he might endure, or how he would face the world. In all his pragmatism, Bill merely wondered, "How will I wear my glasses?"

For nine years, Bill had been fighting off hundreds of cancerous skin lesions that attacked his body, mostly his face. Most people who develop skin cancer get just one or two lesions in their entire lives, typically from having spent too much time in the sun. When people are plagued with hundreds or even thousands of skin lesions, they more than likely have what's called basal cell nevus syndrome, or BCNS.

BCNS is an autosomal dominant disorder. To understand better what this means, here's a quick lesson in genetics: Autosomal refers to a chromosome other than a sex chromosome, so when a disorder has the word *autosomal* in its name, you know it's referring to a condition unrelated to gender. Children inherit two copies of every gene from their parents, one from their mother and one from their father. When a condition is called *dominant*, it means that just one copy of a mutated gene is required to trigger the disorder. So, for example, a parent with an autosomal dominant disorder has one mutated gene and one normal gene. Let's say the other parent's genes are normal. Their child is sure to inherit a normal gene from the unaffected parent, but he or she has a 50 percent chance of inheriting the mutated gene from the parent with the disorder.

Basal cell nevus syndrome is characterized by a predisposition to basal cell lesions, particularly on the face, back, and chest. The trouble with BCNS is twofold: First, depending upon the severity of the disease, the lesions can appear in such vast numbers and so quickly and for so many years that it is physically and emotionally overwhelming to keep up with them. Second, the lesions eat away at the skin and tissue of the affected area, often leaving people who have the syndrome terribly scarred and disfigured. So even if a woman with BCNS has lesions removed from her cheek, for example, and undergoes reconstructive surgery, she may wake up one morning and find another lesion on that same cheek, as well as one on her nose. For some people affected by the syndrome, the lesions fall on them like rain.

People with the syndrome also are predisposed to certain other types of cancers, as well as developmental disorders. Most commonly, individuals with BCNS have bone anomalies — split ribs, for example — and have high foreheads and large heads, a condition known as macrocephaly. The palms of their hands are pitted with tiny holes known as palmar pits, and the soles of their feet often have similar hollows, called plantar pits. They also are highly susceptible to benign, or noncancerous, jaw cysts, found most often in the lower jaw, which is where Bill's nightmare began.

Bill was ten years old when a painful toothache landed him in the dentist's chair, a place where he would subsequently spend much of his adolescence. X-rays revealed a jaw cyst, which would require the skill of an oral surgeon to remove. Never having experienced this before, Bill and his parents had no idea of what to expect. The surgeon sedated Bill with general anesthesia. While under, Bill swallowed copious amounts of blood from the surgery. When he awoke, his gut revolted, violently shooting its contents upward. Bill left a trail of bloody vomit from the oral surgeon's office all the way home, stopping only to take a few shallow breaths and clutch his stomach before the next bout of vomiting began.

By the time Bill was 17, several more jaw cysts had been removed, although each surgery was performed using only Novocain so that he wouldn't be sick afterward. The downside was that the pain following the surgery was tremendous. Somewhere in the middle was the trade-off: being awake during the procedure. Sometimes he would close his eyes, but Bill would usually watch the entire surgery in the reflection of his surgeon's glasses. He felt compelled to look, as though he were driving past a car wreck or watching a horror film with his hands over his eyes, fingers spread just wide enough apart to see the screen.

Pain medication had little or no effect. Bill had no comfort other than his bed, where he'd stay for days afterward in agony. The many surgeries left gaping holes in his upper and lower jaws, eventually destroying all his permanent teeth.

Despite having nearly a dozen jaw cysts in as many years, Bill (and his parents) didn't know the cysts were part of a larger problem, a symptom of a terrible syndrome. Deep inside, though, Bill suspected something was wrong. "These things were happening to me and to no one else that I knew," he says.

The jaw cysts were physically grueling for Bill and heart-wrenching for his mother. "She used to say she felt like she was leading a lamb to slaughter," says Bill of the trips to the surgeon. Even when Bill was an adult, seeing his face wrapped in bandages caused her enormous grief.

She would wonder how Bill seemed to handle the surgeries so well. "There really wasn't another choice," Bill, who is now 61, explains. "It was that or die."

Eventually, Bill chose not to go to the dentist anymore. The jaw cysts stopped developing. Four years later, however, he would enter a new phase of the syndrome.

BCNS IS ALSO KNOWN as Gorlin's syndrome, named for the doctor who first described the spectrum of the disease in 1960. The syndrome is rare; the best estimates peg incidence at about one in 50,000 people in the United States. (Bill thinks of it like this: Imagine being at the Super Bowl and looking around at the crowd. Out of all those people, you'd be the only one with the syndrome.) It's fortunate that the disease is so rare — few people have to endure it — but the flip side is that fewer dollars are available for research. Drug companies aren't interested in developing a cure from which so few people can benefit.

BCNS is genetic, although spontaneous cases do erupt. Between 35 and 50 percent of cases are spontaneous mutations, which essentially means they just happen without a known cause. The chance of an affected individual passing the mutation on to his or her child is

50 percent, and the chance of an affected child having disease severity similar to the parent's is roughly the same. Neither of Bill's parents, both deceased, is thought to have had Gorlin's, nor do his two sisters have it.

People with BCNS are cautioned to avoid unnecessary sun exposure to minimize the risk of acquiring new lesions, although, as Bill says, "I could literally live in a cave and still get them." In addition to his face, the lesions have infiltrated most parts of Bill's body, from the top of his head to the tips of his toes.

In keeping with the typical aspects of the syndrome, Bill was 21 when his first skin lesion appeared; the average age for a basal cell carcinoma to show up on someone affected with the syndrome is 20 years. The lesion appeared as a red, scaly spot on his forehead, about the diameter of a pencil eraser, and it wouldn't go away. Bill finally went to a dermatologist near his hometown of Mount Vernon, New York, just north of the Bronx. The dermatologist, Bill remembers, thought it was odd for someone so young to have a basal cell carcinoma — leading Bill, in hindsight, to believe the doctor may have suspected BCNS.

"I think he knew right away," says Bill, recalling how the dermatologist specifically looked at Bill's palms. However, he added, "If the doctor did know, he never let on."

Over the next year, Bill's dermatologist discovered several more basal cell carcinomas, also called nevi, and removed them, typically using cryosurgery, a method of destroying cells by freezing them. Then, just as suddenly as the first lesion appeared, they stopped. It was as though their commander in chief blew the horn of surrender and the army of red spots beat a hasty retreat. It would be eight years before the lesions would regroup and stage another attack. And this time, it would be a blitzkrieg.

In the meantime, Bill married Diane, the love of his life. He held a stable job as a computer programmer at *Reader's Digest*, where he and Diane first met. It was 1974. Bill and Diane were happily in love, and life looked so promising.

Then the lesions made a comeback, as though they were waiting for a time when Bill's guard was down. Their timing was perfect. He was settling into Diane's apartment and getting used to his new role as a husband when the first lesion appeared, pitching camp in Bill's ear. He tried to ignore the lesion, but it grew larger and larger. Eventually, the lesion broke open and began to ooze pus. Bill finally sought the help of another dermatologist, who asked all the right questions and immediately diagnosed basal cell nevus syndrome.

In that pre-Internet era, medical information was hard to come by, and getting information about a rare disease was harder still. The average family physician might never even see a cancerous skin lesion in his or her entire career.

The dermatologist suggested that Bill seek genetic counseling to confirm the diagnosis and to see whether the disease could be passed on to his children. If it was hereditary, Bill and Diane, married just two years, would be faced with the difficult decision of whether to start a family of their own. They needed to learn how great the risk was of their children inheriting the syndrome, and based on that risk, they would need to decide where their comfort level fell. For instance, were they comfortable if there was a 70 percent chance that their children would be unaffected? What if the odds decreased to 50 percent? Was that too much of a risk? Where would they draw the line? And if the syndrome was hereditary, could their children have it worse than Bill did?

Alone, Bill consulted a genetic counselor, and to his two most pressing questions, he received an affirmative response. Yes, he did indeed have the syndrome and, yes, it could be passed on to his children. The risk was 50 percent.

Fifty-fifty, the flip of a coin. The odds were even. That seemed too large a gamble, and Bill wasn't much of a gambling man. Hearing the geneticist say that he had a 50 percent chance of passing on a serious and painful disease to his child was dizzying. He couldn't do this to a child, not after everything he'd been through himself: cysts, planted in his jaw like land mines, and lesions — the hundreds and hundreds of poisonous lesions — that grew deep within his tissues and erupted out of his skin, stealing his face, little by little… How could he take that risk? How could he knowingly pass on that legacy?

But it was too much information too late. Diane was already expecting a child. At the moment Bill got the news, he thought of Diane, nurturing the tiny life inside her and not yet knowing what he knew. She was at home, thinking about what color to paint the baby's room, washing all the new baby clothes, and choosing an outfit for the baby to wear home from the hospital. Diane loved children and was eager to have a whole houseful. To Diane, this baby, her first, would be just that — the first of many.

Sitting in the geneticist's office, Bill made "a unilateral decision" not to have any more children. His heart ached at the thought of telling Diane, who, despite the evidence and the risk, would feel differently.

After learning the news, Diane remembers thinking that everything would be all right. "I looked forward to having our son and that was that," she says. Besides, at the time, the only significant manifestations she and Bill associated with the syndrome were jaw cysts; the basal cell lesions seemed secondary and manageable. Bill had had his last jaw cyst surgery about ten years before he met Diane. Although she understood the cysts were painful, she hadn't truly experienced that aspect of the syndrome. To her mind, if her children inherited the syndrome and had a few jaw cysts, she could live with it. Diane was willing to take the risk.

The procedure to remove the lesion from Bill's ear was far more involved than what could be accomplished in a dermatologist's office. He was referred to Memorial Sloan-Kettering Cancer Center in New York City and was seen by physicians from several different departments. They, in turn, referred Bill to New York University Medical Center. There, Bill consulted with Dr. Michael J. Albom, a clinical professor of dermatology at the Ronald O. Perelman Department of Dermatology and surgeon who specialized in Mohs micrographic surgery, reconstructive surgery, and dermatological surgery. He successfully removed the lesion in Bill's ear.

Basal cell carcinoma—absent the syndrome—is one of the most common types of skin cancer; another is squamous cell carcinoma. Typically, lesions are caught early and removed without a problem. Most people who develop a lesion will have only one or two in their entire life.

All skin cancers begin on the surface of the skin and spread downward and sideways, much the way water reacts when you water a plant, moving outward and down toward the plant's roots. As with a plant, cancerous lesions have "roots" that cannot be seen from the skin's surface. Therefore, to make sure the entire lesion is removed, the surgeon often must dig deep. How deep? Unless the surgeon is using Mohs micrographic surgery, he or she is only guessing.

Tedious and time-consuming, Mohs micrographic surgery involves several steps. The first two steps are to scrape away the cancerous lesion, using a curette, and to surgically remove an additional layer of tissue surrounding and including the scraped area.

"This tissue is placed on a gauze pad or petri dish and is oriented physically in the same direction as its original position on the person," explains Dr. Albom. "The surgically removed tissue is subdivided into multiple smaller segments, and each cut edge of the segments is color-coded with dyes."

The next step is to create an anatomical map, upon which a diagram of the patient's exact surgical site is hand drawn. The diagram on the map is color-coded identically to the tissue segments that were just removed from the patient, says Dr. Albom, who explains, "This compulsive technique ensures that the precise location and orientation of the removed tissue will be identical to the drawn map." Having this anatomical map is crucial to the surgeon in order to determine the exact location of the cancerous and noncancerous tissue.

In the Mohs laboratory, the tissue is dipped in liquid nitrogen for freezing and comes out looking like a mini-snowball. The snowball is placed onto the equivalent of a meat slicer and cut into super-thin slices (six microns or so, thinner than pencil shavings). The slices are placed on glass slides, stained, and viewed under a microscope to determine whether cancerous cells are present. Checking the edges of the tissue is crucial, because if cancerous cells are seen on the edge, the surgeon must go wider or deeper when removing the next layer of tissue. If any cancerous cells are observed, the Mohs surgeon marks this information on the anatomical map. The surgeon returns to the patient with the map and removes another layer of skin in the area where the cancerous cells remain. The process is repeated, typically taking hours, until the surgeon sounds the "all clear." Once the tissue is free of cancerous cells, the process ends.

The technique is named after its pioneer, Dr. Frederic Mohs, who wanted to spare as much healthy tissue as possible in his skin cancer patients while at the same time ensuring that all the cancer was removed. By surgically cutting away only the layers of tissue that are cancerous, healthy tissue is spared and the surgeon is confident that no cancerous cells are left behind.

Using the traditional excision technique, the surgeon is never absolutely sure that all the cancerous tissue is excised. The surgeon relies on the hospital pathologist to check the margins (edges) of the surgically removed tissue for cancerous cells, and the pathologist examines only a tiny percentage of the margins. Some estimates are 1 percent to 5 percent of the total, says Dr. Albom. "This methodology is not nearly as compulsive as the 100 percent margin analysis done with Mohs surgery," he says.

Mohs surgery was introduced in the 1930s but didn't become the standard of care for complex skin cancers until the mid-1990s. Its success rate is outstanding: 99 percent cure rate for patients with basal cell carcinoma and 97 percent for patients with squamous cell carcinoma.

Of course, there is a direct correlation between the procedure's success and the skill of the Mohs surgeon. In the United States today, there are approximately 800 Mohs surgeons who have been trained by the fellowship programs sponsored by the American College of Mohs Micrographic Surgery and Cutaneous Oncology. The organization requires years of rigorous clinical training. Although alternative programs exist for dermatologists and their histotechnologists (the persons preparing Mohs microscopic slides) to learn Mohs micrographic surgery, they offer minimal training.

"A qualified Mohs surgeon must be able to treat a spectrum of patients, including those with very aggressive tumors in critical anatomic locations — especially around the eyes, for example," says Dr. Albom. The histotechnologist must also be expertly trained; a Mohs surgeon cannot interpret slides with accuracy unless the technician's work is outstanding.

Although the technique is designed to spare tissue, Mohs surgery can still leave a scar. A cancerous lesion the size of a small pimple — particularly on the nose — can infiltrate surrounding tissue enough so that, following Mohs surgery, the wound is the size of a silver dollar.

There is no way to predict accurately the true size of any skin cancer just by visually inspecting it, says Dr. Albom, who has been practicing for more than 30 years and sees many patients with complex problems in his private practice in New York. Several factors determine whether a small lesion may actually be the tip of the iceberg.

"Certain histologic tumor types, such as morpheiform or infiltrative basal cell carcinomas, can widely invade the skin and sometimes the underlying deeper structures," he explains. "Patients with recurrent disease or treatment failures, or those who have had previous radiation treatments for conditions like acne and hirsutism, can also be among those who present with seemingly small lesions that, in reality, are much larger."

Patients with BCNS, like Bill, also can walk into their doctor's office with what appears to be a tiny spot on their nose and leave with what must feel like an abyss. Still, using the Mohs procedure, the amount of tissue spared compared with traditional excision is significant, and there's little question that the cancer is gone.

SOON AFTER THE LESION was removed from Bill's ear, his usual dermatologist died and he neglected to find a new one. When Bill developed a serious lesion on his right thigh, his primary care physician insisted that he consult a dermatologist, but Bill wasn't persuaded. He'd had enough of doctors, especially dermatologists. He felt he needed some time off. His "sabbatical" would last for nearly a decade.

As the lesion on Bill's thigh grew worse, a tiny dot appeared on his face. The dot turned into two dots, which then turned into four dots and then eight. The dots appeared overnight, just as mysteriously as crop circles in the English countryside. Numbering into the dozens, the lesions formed dark patches across Bill's nose, spreading to his cheek and toward his mouth like black mold in a damp basement.

Diane begged Bill to see a doctor, especially when the lesions appeared ready to take over his entire face. "My God, it was like a huge scab," she says, but he refused, and soon she stopped asking.

Finally, he consulted with a dermatologist, who gave him the shocking news that he probably would lose his nose. "If you had waited longer," the dermatologist told him, "you might have lost your eyes, too."

His dermatologist recommended two Mohs surgeons to Bill, one of whom was Dr. Albom, the same surgeon who'd done the work on his ear years before. Bill met with Dr. Albom, who acknowledged that he had a major job on his hands and that in all likelihood Bill would lose his nose.

"It was a shock," says Dr. Albom upon seeing Bill again, this time with massive lesions covering the center of his face and looking very different from how he had looked ten years earlier. "It was absolutely unbelievable," he says, noting that Bill hadn't truly manifested the syndrome until that time.

"I kept making stupid excuses about why I didn't want to go," recalls Bill. Looking back, he cannot explain why he didn't seek help earlier, but one can imagine that he was simply tired of going to the doctor and afraid of what he might hear if he went.

Every time someone with BCNS develops a lesion, which can be frequently, it means a trip to the doctor and a surgical procedure. (According to the 2004–05 *Guinness World Records*, Charles Jensen of Chester, South Dakota, underwent 970 surgical procedures, the most operations ever endured, to remove lesions associated with basal cell nevus syndrome. The procedures took place over a 40-year period, mainly at Mayo Clinic in Rochester, Minnesota.) People with the syndrome sometimes require months to years of treatment and continual care, says Dr. Albom, who manages more than a half-dozen patients with BCNS. "It's a pretty miserable disease. Few people have the stamina to follow through for years with a long-term treatment plan to keep this chronic disease under as much control as possible," he adds.

People with the syndrome become fearful of looking in the mirror, afraid of detecting one of those wretched spots, whose diminutive size belies its capacity for destruction. They grow tired of facing the enemy over and over again. Each battle leaves them more scarred than the last, and the distinction of winning the battle doesn't leave them feeling all that satisfied.

For these people, however, denial is an enemy they can't afford to have. A lesion is like the red laser dot of a sniper's rifle. Once the disease, like a sniper, sets its sights, it doesn't often retreat.

Dr. Albom knew he could help Bill and recommended involving Dr. William Shaw (now retired), who was then chief of Plastic Surgery at Bellevue Hospital in New York City. Bill immediately felt at ease. He held Dr. Albom in the highest esteem and does to this day, considering him a cherished friend. Additionally, about a week prior, he'd seen a local television news broadcast featuring Dr. Shaw. A woman had been pinned beneath a fallen crane, which crushed her legs. Dr. Shaw was in charge of the woman's reconstructive surgery, and he appeared to be skilled, confident, and trustworthy. Together, Drs. Albom and Shaw were exactly what Bill needed.

The doctors met with Bill to devise a treatment and recovery plan. Bill would be hospitalized for several days while the lesions and tissue of his nose were surgically removed, one layer at a time, to minimize the amount of tissue removal. Still, Dr. Albom was certain that Bill would lose his entire nose.

Bill was 38 when the first of the many Mohs surgeries began on his nose. (He would be 43 by the time the surgeries were finished and his nose was reconstructed.) His wife and son, Billy, who was about nine at the time, were at home and unable to visit much. Bill weathered his surgery alone. Perhaps because of adequate medications, he didn't feel much pain during the Mohs procedures, which, because of the number of lesions, ended up taking weeks.

"I just went along with the program," he says, recalling a sense of numbness and surrender. He never inquired as to how much of his nose had been removed on any particular day, and he wasn't interested in seeing the result of the surgery until it presented itself one day quite by accident.

Bill had gotten out of bed to use the restroom. While he was in the bathroom, the bandage came loose and slipped down, revealing the extent of the surgery. He turned to the bathroom mirror to adjust the bandage and was struck by what he saw — or, rather, by what he didn't see. Bill's entire nose was gone, and so was a large chunk of flesh beneath his right eye and a good part of his upper lip on the right side. From his eyebrows to his chin, his face was more or less flat. Beneath the complex skin graft molded to his flesh, he could see a single bone running down the center of the space where his nose used to be. His hands clutched the sides of the cool porcelain sink as he stared into the graft's grid-like pattern.

"I remember thinking I could be in a horror movie without makeup. I literally almost threw up."

He stumbled back to the hospital bed. After that, whenever the bandage became loose, Bill would fix it without the benefit of a mirror or ring the nurse-call bell for help.

BEFORE BILL COULD BE released from the hospital, Diane had to learn some caregiving skills. One of Bill's nurses showed her the wound and explained how to change the dressings, what kinds of things to watch for, such as infection, and what kinds of things to expect. If Diane was bothered by the sight of Bill's face or having to change his dressings, she didn't show it. "I loved Bill, and I hated to see him go through this. But we were going to do this together," Diane says.

Bill was happy to be back home with Diane and Billy. And Diane was eager to help get Bill back on his feet. Although they'd both been through so much, it seemed as though the worst was behind them. Little Billy was healthy, Bill was recovering — he'd learned his lesson about avoiding the dermatologist — and Diane had her husband back home.

Diane's main job was to change the dressings on Bill's face regularly. Using the technique she'd learned at the hospital, she went about changing his dressing for the first time. "I was trying to be so gentle to get the bandage off, but it was clinging," she says. The dressing had gotten stuck on a scab on Bill's cheek. When Diane tugged harder to remove the dressing, the scab ripped away and let loose a torrent of bright red blood, pulsing furiously from an artery in Bill's face.

"The blood just gushed all over the place," says Diane. She ran to get towels and tried to stop the blood flow with pressure to Bill's cheek. After soaking several bath towels, Diane rushed to the linen closet and grabbed beach towels. In no time, those were soaked with blood. At that point, Bill began to get nervous.

Diane had been entrusted with Bill's care, and now he was lying on the couch, awash in blood. It was her job to care for him, to change his dressings. He'd been through so much already, living through major surgery and a raging infection that nearly killed him, and now he was going to die on the couch.

The hospital was four miles from their apartment. Diane wiped away the sweat and hair from her eyes, smearing her husband's blood across her forehead. She needed to get to the hospital quickly or Bill was going to bleed to death.

"I couldn't get him out of the house fast enough to get him to the hospital," says Diane. "I almost had to carry him to the car."

Diane raced Bill to the hospital emergency room. The four miles seemed like 20. "I thought he was going to die on me," she says. "I was scared to death."

At the hospital, the emergency room staff was able to get Bill's bleeding under control. Because he'd lost so much blood, he spent the night at the hospital for observation, returning home the next day to Diane, who resumed her caregiving duties even more cautiously.

IN 1986, JUST ABOUT the time Bill had the rhinectomy, his son, then ten, was diagnosed with a jaw cyst — a clear sign he'd inherited the syndrome. If it weren't that Bill half-expected his son to inherit the syndrome — after all, the risk was 50/50 — the news would have felt like a sucker punch. Instead it felt inevitable, the way it feels when your foot lands in a patch of slick mud and pulls you forward, upending your body.

Still, "It just about killed me," he says. Each time he'd take his son to the oral surgeon, his own mother's words — "leading a lamb to the slaughter" — echoed in his ears. Bill had suffered from the excruciating pain of the jaw cyst surgeries, and now he ached for his young son who shared the same fate.

Although it broke Diane's heart to watch her son suffer, she says she would have had more children if Bill had agreed. "I begged him," she recalls. "I was willing to take the chance. It was easier for me because I didn't have the syndrome."

Years later, Bill would look back to the day his son was born and realize that the signs that he'd inherited the disease were there. At the time, though, they hadn't known about all the signs. For instance, Billy was born with a very large head, so large that the obstetrician thought the baby might have hydrocephalus, or "water on the brain." Results from a CT scan performed when he was just a few days old came back negative; thus, his large head had remained a mystery to the medical staff, as well as to his parents.

Despite newer, more powerful pain medications, Billy's nine jaw cyst surgeries were no easier than his father's had been. The pain was extreme, and every surgery required an overnight hospital stay.

"Through the years, my father has endured a tremendous amount of pain and aggravation from Gorlin's, but I admire the way he has handled it every step of the way," says Billy, who is in his early thirties. "I've looked up to him for that, and that is what kept me going through some of the toughest times that I've personally gone through with this syndrome."

Because the syndrome is hereditary, Billy and his wife struggled with the decision of whether to start their own family. Should they have a child and take that 50/50 risk? Although Billy wanted a brother or sister when he was younger, he understands why he is an only child. He and his wife chose adoption, and in 2008 welcomed baby Brianna into their lives.

Billy's first basal cell lesion appeared in 2005, just weeks after his dentist suspected another jaw cyst on an X-ray. Much to everyone's relief, the suspicious spot seen on the X-ray turned out to be scar tissue. However, the lesion didn't go away with medication, and Billy underwent a Mohs procedure to have it removed. Since then, he's found another lesion on his nose.

ABOUT TWO YEARS AFTER Bill's rhinectomy, it was time to begin the reconstruction process.

Diane recalls Bill coming home from seeing Dr. Shaw and saying, "You're not going to believe what they want to do to me."

To rebuild Bill's nose, Dr. Shaw needed a reasonable amount of Bill's own skin. However, in persons with BCNS, most of their skin is predisposed to developing basal cell lesions, so finding a suitable "donor" area on their body is a challenge. Dr. Shaw chose Bill's inner forearm, because it's a spot that typically gets little sun exposure and therefore had the lowest probability of being predisposed to developing cancerous lesions.

"I told Dr. Shaw, 'Look, you're not going to know if this skin is disease-free,' but we took the chance," says Dr. Albom.

For some rhinectomy patients, a prosthetic nose is a more reasonable option. However, in Bill's case, Drs. Shaw and Albom didn't feel it was a good choice for two reasons. For one, 20 years ago, many nasal prosthetics didn't look that good. "The aesthetic skill wasn't readily available. Few people had the expertise to make a prosthetic nose that had a natural appearance," Dr. Albom says. Second, keeping a nasal prosthesis securely in place was tricky. Adhesives often didn't hold well enough. For example, wearers ran the risk of having their nose suddenly fall off their face. Another solution required drilling holes in the facial bone and attaching the prosthesis with magnets. Although this option gave wearers a better sense of security, the risk of bone infection, which could lead to more serious problems, was a real threat. Drs. Albom and Shaw simply couldn't predict the potential negative consequences related to a prosthesis. After serious consideration, they determined that reconstructive surgery was the best option for Bill.

Dr. Shaw, who later was the chief of Plastic Surgery at UCLA before retiring, inserted a skin expander into Bill's left inner forearm. The expander is nothing more than a balloon that is filled very slowly over time with saline solution, allowing the skin beneath it to expand gradually, the way pregnancy expands a woman's belly. The extra tissue created by the skin expansion is then used as a microvascular free flap; in Bill's case, it was used to rebuild his nose.

Months later, once the tissue on Bill's forearm was stretched enough, Dr. Shaw fashioned a new nose for Bill right on his arm. Cartilage was taken from Bill's rib cage to help shape the tip of his new nose. So that the nose would heal into its new shape, it had to remain attached to the blood supply on Bill's arm. So his nose, complete with a bridge and two nostrils, stayed on his arm for several more months, protected on four sides by a small cardboard box, which was covered with gauze and affixed with surgical tape.

"It was radical, the way he did it," says Bill, recalling his amazement when he looked at his new nose for the first time. "I wondered how on earth the nose on my arm was going to be transplanted onto my face."

During the time that Bill's nose was "growing" on his arm, he'd had several appointments with other physicians. "The doctors were in awe. They were just in awe," recalls Diane. But Bill, being Bill, took it in stride. "He made a lot of jokes about it," says Diane. "He'd say, 'My arm is sneezing!' It was quite funny most of the time."

Several months later, Dr. Shaw transplanted Bill's new nose from his arm to his face. The procedure took about eight hours and was accomplished without complication.

AFTER THE RHINECTOMY and reconstruction, Bill was still battling the onslaught of lesions. He learned of a clinical trial at Roswell Park Cancer Institute in Buffalo to test photodynamic therapy, or PDT. The trial involved injecting a drug into Bill's bloodstream that would attach itself to cancerous cells. A few days after the injection, the physician would destroy the lesions using lasers specially designed to target the cancerous cells. The PDT treatments themselves were painless, but days later, the sites would "hurt like hell," says Bill. "Like cigarette burns."

Bill's current dermatologist, whom he sees every three months, treats his basal cell lesions with electrodesiccation, or "scrape and burn." The treatment is quick and leaves only small scars — a far cry from the cigarette-like burns and loss of facial features he's had to endure. Dermatologists also are using a variety of topical chemicals such as Efudex and newer topical immunomodulators to boost the immune system. Aldara (imiquimod) induces interferon, which is a chemical the body naturally produces as a defense against various stresses. Retinoids, which are a vitamin A derivative, have shown some promise, too, in treating basal cell lesions.

For Bill, the torrent of lesions has slowed in recent years, perhaps because of his age. The body tends to change in mysterious ways as it gets older. One hopes that after one spends so long in a downpour, the clouds might recede and the rain dwindle to a drizzle.

BILL'S NASAL RECONSTRUCTION, undergone more than 20 years ago, is still a success. He has total feeling throughout most of his nasal area, lacking some feeling only at the base, where his nose meets his upper lip. This lack of sensation presents a problem only in the winter, when he cannot feel his nose running.

Naturally, his face is scarred from the various surgeries and treatments to remove the lesions. Some of his facial skin appears pitted and pulled, the way skin sometimes looks after having been burned. Most people assume he was in a fire.

Still, Bill is a confident, kind man with a healthy self-image, so long as he doesn't look too hard at himself. He doesn't particularly like to see photographs of himself. Once, standing in front of a three-sided mirror in a dressing room, he caught a glimpse of his profile. The mirrors offered Bill an entirely different view from what he'd seen by looking directly into a mirror. He couldn't believe what he saw. "I was shocked," he says. Now he simply avoids mirrors.

BCNS AND THE EFFECT it has had on Bill's appearance contributed to his and Diane's later marital trouble, he believes. He felt she couldn't cope with other people's reactions to how he looked. "Diane was bothered when people would stare," Bill says. "It didn't bother me as much. I just shrugged it off or didn't even notice it."

It wasn't until recently that Diane came to terms with how she felt then. "I have to admit, I hated going out in public with him," she confesses. "We'd go out in public and people would stare. It bothered me tremendously."

Finally, they stopped going out as a couple. The time they spent together diminished and their conversations grew shorter. Their increasing disconnectedness made Diane feel lonely. She wanted to share a normal life with Bill inside and outside their home, but she couldn't get past the gawking eyes, the stink of sulfurous stares.

Then one day, Diane came to Bill and said she didn't want to be married anymore. Bill was devastated, but he didn't know what to do to keep her. In 1994, after 20 years of marriage, they divorced.

TO BILL, HAVING BCNS means that nothing is normal. "You can't count on anything," he says, "but you have to think positive." BCNS stole precious things from Bill: a large part of his face, his marriage, and a certain amount of self-confidence. Yet he never asked, "Why me?" On the contrary, Bill insists that the syndrome has made him the person he is today.

"I like who I am, and I wouldn't be that person had I not gone through what I did," he says.

Prior to recently retiring, Bill worked for an organization that helps men who are recovering from alcohol and drug addiction. The work was satisfying, because he was truly making a difference in people's lives. Perhaps it's because the focus was on others and not on him.

Because of the basal cell nevus syndrome, Bill knows what it's like to feel different from other people. He understands how it feels to have a disease like alcohol or chemical dependency take over your life, tear at your self-esteem, and destroy your family. The men he saw every day accepted him for who he is and how he looks. They didn't stare at him or judge him because he looks different from them. When Bill smiled and offered an outstretched hand, someone accepted it and smiled right back.

⚙

CHAPTER 2

what is a face?

Cracked pots allow the treasure to shine forth.

— Jim Watkins

L
IKE SNOWFLAKES AND FINGERPRINTS, no two faces are exactly alike. Even identical twins have slight differences in their appearance, allowing those closest to them to tell them apart with little more than a sideways glance. When you consider that a face has fewer than a dozen components — eyes, ears, nose, mouth, eyebrows, forehead, chin, and cheeks — the fact that every face looks different is astonishing. How is it possible?

The answer is more than skin deep. Variations in bone structure, muscle and skin tone, and tissue thickness account for the uniqueness of billions of people. If you take two images of the same person and slightly alter the shape of the head, size of the ears, or width of the eyes on one image, the difference becomes striking.

Take noses. Even minor deviations in size, length, width, the degree of the bend, and downturn make a difference. Is the tip of the nose sharp or bulbous? To what degree? Is it covered with freckles or redder than surrounding features? What about the size of the nostrils? Do they flare?

Just a slight variation in structure or tissue placement can change the appearance of a face. Plastic surgeons and their patients have known this for years. An eyebrow lift can turn back time, a chin implant can provide missing symmetry, and a nose job can brighten an entire face. What's interesting is that the differences often are so slight, we hardly notice them. This is why a person who recently had a face-lift might hear, "You look different. Did you change your hairstyle?"

Notice how color affects a person's appearance. Skin tone, hair color, and eye color help define what a person looks like. Think how different a fair-skinned woman might look after vacationing in Mexico for a week. Her hair might be lighter, her skin darker, and she might even have fewer wrinkles, temporarily, from being so relaxed. The presence or absence of hair dramatically changes how someone looks, too. A man who typically sports a beard and mustache looks much different when he's clean-shaven. Fine nuances such as the distance between the base of the nose and the lips, the length of the chin, or the shape of the eyebrows also contribute to a person's unique appearance.

It's easy to say you know what someone looks like, but it's much tougher to describe a person in sufficient detail to make someone else understand. Victims of crime who sit with the police sketch artist are proof of this. Almond-shaped eyes, olive skin, pointy nose, thin lips, ears close to his head. Give that description to three artists, and they'll all come back with different renderings.

Separately, our parts are just that: parts. But together, they're even more than how we look. They help shape how we face the world: with confidence, with hesitation, or with fear of rejection.

THE FACE IS PRINCIPALLY made up of three parts: the brain and basicranium (the bottom or "floor" of the skull), the airway region, and the oral region. Dr. Mark Hans is a professor and head of the Department of Orthodontics at Case Western Reserve University's School of Dental Medicine in Cleveland. In a book he co-authored, Dr. Hans theorized that although the regions develop according to their own timetables, development is programmed in such a way as to create a final proportional balance in the face. For example, a baby's face has a small nasal and oral area to match the size of its lungs and pulmonary function. Perfect balance doesn't truly occur, however, which accounts for the variety of faces we meet every day.

Of the 14 bones in the face, the lower jawbone (inferior maxillary bone or mandible, from the Latin *mandere*, which means "to chew") is the largest and strongest. The upper jawbone is actually a combination of two bones, called superior maxillary bones, and forms the second-largest bone of the face. The two cheekbones (zygomatic bones) make up the floor of the eye sockets and the sockets' outer wall. The smallest, most fragile bones of the face are the two lachrymal bones. The size of fingernails, they're found inside the wall of the eye sockets. The bridge of the nose is formed by the confluence of two nasal bones that rest side by side. Two palate bones are found between the two halves of the upper jawbone and help complete the roof of the mouth, the floor and outer wall of the nasal area, and the floor of the eye sockets. Along each side of the nose is an inferior turbinated bone. These bones, which are spongy and curled like a scroll, serve as canals for veins and arteries. Finally, the vomer, located behind the nasal bones, is a single bone that forms the septum, or dividing wall.

Through their shape and size, the 14 facial bones and eight bones of the cranium influence a person's appearance. For example, the width and thickness of the frontal bone will dictate the shape of the forehead. It may be long and narrow, contributing to an "egghead" look; short and wide, giving the head a squat look; or dozens of variations in between.

Ten groups of facial muscles control a wide range of movement and allow us to show hundreds of expressions, from happiness and surprise to disappointment and curiosity. The muscles around the eyes and mouth are a series of concentric circles that resemble bull's-eyes. Each muscle group has between one and seven muscles, with the most belonging to the nasal and eye regions. The eyes and eyelids require sophisticated musculature to hold the orbit, or eyeball, in place and to support the complex movements associated with vision.

Twelve categories of cranial nerves are responsible for all sorts of facial expressions and sensory functions. Specific nerves control eye movement and sight. Thus, injury to the third cranial nerve, which controls most of the muscles to the eye, may result in ptosis, or drooping of the upper eyelid, among other things. Injury to the fourth cranial nerve may prevent the eye from looking downward and outward. Other nerves control our senses of hearing, smell, and taste. Speaking, smiling, and chewing would be impossible if not for the cranial nerves.

Blood to the head and neck is supplied by the common carotid artery, which branches off into two sections right below the chin. One branch, the internal artery, supplies blood to the cranial cavity. The other branch feeds blood to the head and face. Called the external artery, it runs deep under the lower jaw, then climbs up and over the jaw, up through the cheek and alongside the nose, and ends deep behind the eye, its branches spreading across the face like a perfect specimen of sea fan coral.

"FACE FIRST" IS THE TITLE of an undergraduate seminar Dr. Hans led at Case Western Reserve University. He says the class was the culmination of two watershed events in his life. The first was the "huge personality transformation" he witnessed in patients following orthodontia treatment. The second was an observation during a visit to Paris. At the Louvre, he noticed that all the visitors wanted their photographs taken with the statue of Venus de Milo. This fascination with Venus appeared to cross cultural lines; it didn't matter that Venus was an ancient Greek beauty. She appeared to represent ideal beauty to all.

The "Face First" seminar explored six face-related themes that ranged from identity and beauty to facial communication and deformity. One session of the seminar was titled "Eye of the Beholder," after an episode from the 1960s television series *The Twilight Zone*. In the episode, a young woman is shown in a hospital room, her head and face bandaged. She had undergone surgery to correct her facial disfiguration. The room is full of doctors and nurses, but the viewer doesn't see them — just hears their voices. In the last scene, her face is unwrapped and, to everyone's horror, including her own, she looks just as she did before the surgery. The camera focuses on her face, which is beautiful by our standards, and then pans to the team of doctors and nurses, who all have faces like those of wild boars.

And then, there is a well-known folktale about a child who has become separated from his mother. The little boy is crying because he is lost. When asked what his mother looks like, he says, "My mother is the most beautiful woman in the world." All the men in town bring the most attractive women back to the boy, one after another, but none of them is his mother. One day, a cart pulls into town with a rather plain-looking woman, wearing a babushka to cover her unruly hair. She looks around desperately. Suddenly she hears her son cry, "Mother!"

Finally, mother and son are reunited, and the townsfolk smile at one another knowingly, muttering, "Ah, yes, the most beautiful woman in the world."

The eye of the beholder aside, one way of measuring beauty or attractiveness in many things is symmetry. A mathematical equation that retains its form, no matter how it is transformed (the equation for a sphere is an example), is considered beautiful by mathematicians because of its symmetry. Cognitive scientists, in what they call the laws of good form, posit that we need to see things in an orderly manner as a way of making sense from chaos. Hence our innate attraction to things symmetrical.

Phi, or divine proportion, is the mathematical ratio for beauty: 1:1.618. The ratio applies to dimensions of facial features, such as width of the face to length of the face; width of the mouth to width of the cheek; width of the nose to width of the cheek; and width of the nose to width of the mouth. So, for example, if the width of the face from cheek to cheek is five inches, the length of the face should be 8.09 inches to be in divine proportion.

That relatively few of us meet the standards of divine proportion doesn't deter television and advertising from bombarding us with images of how we should look, fueling our feelings of inadequacy. The messages are insidious; they've contributed to consumers' demand for medical science to fix even the slightest imperfections, and extreme-makeover reality shows are all the rage. In 2004, China crowned its first Miss Plastic Surgery. The winner, only 22, underwent Botox injections to smooth her features and had cosmetic surgery to widen her eyes and slim her cheeks and waist.

"In defense of people who choose to undergo cosmetic surgery," counters Dr. Andrew Jacono, a facial plastic and reconstructive surgeon in New York, "when a person looks better, they will typically take better care of themselves," adding that any improvement in overall health is a positive change. Dr. Jacono embarked upon a career in plastic surgery as a result of a third-grade classmate's experience with a cleft lip. "She felt ostracized," he says, because of the stigma associated with looking outside of the norm. Like most people, she had a desire to fit in. Those who don't resemble the norm because of a craniofacial condition and those who think they don't measure up to some established standard of beauty or attractiveness share a similar sense of unworthiness, he says.

How we view our physical selves influences us in many ways. A study conducted at Stanford University in Palo Alto, California, found that people's behavior was affected by the appearance of the cartoon images, or avatars, used to represent them in an online game. Half the people in the first group were assigned avatars that were tall; the other half were given avatars that were short. In the second group, half the people were given avatars with more attractive faces than the other half. All the players had less than one minute to "acquaint" themselves with their avatars before playing the virtual game, which involved negotiating money. People with the taller avatars negotiated more aggressively than the group with shorter avatars, and people with the less attractive avatars stood farther away from the more attractive ones. Online behavior was unaffected by what these individuals looked like in real life. Their behavior was solely dependent on their online image, and that it was influenced so quickly is astonishing.

The way we feel about faces and what faces mean to us are naturally expressed in our language. The English language is full of idioms that use the word *face* to refer to identity. "Do you remember that guy we used to work with? You know, what's-his-face?" What's-his-face is another term for what's-his-name, which is really just another form of identity; we identify ourselves closely by our names and our faces. If someone seems to have two separate identities, we might say he is two-faced. Someone who is in your face is physically or figuratively too close. To get face time with someone is to actually see and communicate with that person.

Dignity, which is closely connected to identity, can be communicated by referring to the face: To be ashamed or disgraced is to have egg on your face, to fall on your face, or to lose face. Pride can be restored by putting on a brave face or a game face so that one can, it is hoped, save face.

Because the human face is so closely related to identity, the face gets described more often than any other body part. Unfavorable comparisons abound: a face that could stop a clock, a face like thunder, a face like a bulldog chewing a wasp, a face like the back of a bus, a face like a fiddle, and a face like an unmade bed. Such insults! But the worst kind of insult, no matter what it is, feels like a slap in the face.

WHEN A CHILD IS BORN with a craniofacial defect, we attempt to establish the cause. Today we know that some craniofacial conditions are attributed to genetic defects passed down from generation to generation. More often than not, however, the exact cause is unknown. Even if the abnormality has a genetic basis, it may be a new onset; no one else in the family had the abnormality, so the new case is the family's first. Years ago, people explained birth defects in ways that made rational sense to them, often looking around their environment to make a connection to the defect.

Joseph Merrick, better known as the Elephant Man, attributed his disfigurement to his mother being terribly frightened by a circus elephant during a fair. Though the story was never confirmed, it was said that Joseph's mother, Mary Jane, was nearly trampled by an elephant that was allowed to walk the town streets as an advertisement for the fair. Pushed inadvertently into the elephant's path by the crowd of townspeople, Mary Jane, who was lame, barely moved quickly enough to avoid being crushed to death. About six months pregnant at the time, she was so traumatized by the incident, so the story goes, that her unborn child was imprinted with the likes of an elephant.

Belief in maternal imprinting has a long recorded history. It was thought that any longing, desire, and especially fear a mother might experience while pregnant could mark her unborn baby. The ancient Greeks believed that if a pregnant woman gazed upon pleasant objects, such as artwork, and listened to beautiful music, her child would be born fair. On the other hand, if a wild animal startled a mother, her child might be born disfigured. If she ate too many strawberries, her child might be born with a strawberry-colored birthmark, and spilling coffee or tea on herself might result in a dark-colored birthmark on the baby. Sixteenth-century physician Ambroise Paré suggested that a mother's imagination affected her unborn child and wrote that maternal impression was one of the 13 causes of birth defects in children.

Sprites and evil spirits also were considered a source of birth defects in children. In European folklore, babies born with a physical defect or mental retardation were thought to be the offspring of elves, fairies, or other types of subhuman creatures. Called changelings, these babies were believed to have been substituted for the parents' real children. In some cultures, the changelings were revered and considered good fortune, but in most, they were treated poorly in an attempt to force the fairies to return the stolen children. After Christianity took hold, evil spirits and sometimes the devil himself were considered responsible for stealing healthy babies and replacing them with deformed ones as punishment for the sins of the parents.

An 18th-century obstetrician-anatomist named William Hunter

helped discount the theory of maternal imprinting by questioning his pregnant patients about any emotional trauma they had endured since their babies' conception. Unable to link subsequent birth defects with reported emotional distress, the theory began to lose steam. Dr. Hunter did note, however, that when a birth defect was present, the mother could easily recall the emotional trauma that caused it.

The belief in maternal imprinting made sense to people who could not otherwise make sense of something as traumatic as a serious birth defect or even a modest birthmark. Human nature demands that we try to explain every event, assigning responsibility or blame. Random events, such as spontaneous genetic mutations, leave us searching for an answer to "why?" even though there may be no answer or the answer is "just because." The belief in any superstition is a result of our inability to accept that events can be random. Why else would a pitcher take pains not to step on the third-base line when leaving the mound? Why would a burly, tattooed Harley rider hang a dainty brass bell from the bottom of his bike? (Answer: The bell scares away evil road gremlins that cause motorcycles to break down.) Protecting ourselves from random events with rituals or talismans allows us to feel in control of a chaotic world, which is why the theory of maternal imprinting held fast throughout the 19th century and remains, even today, in some parts of the world.

Dr. John Mulliken, professor of surgery at Harvard Medical School and director of the Craniofacial Centre at Children's Hospital Boston, has written about vascular birthmarks in folklore, noting that the word *birthmark* itself is nearly an indictment of the mother. In other languages, the same is true. In German, for example, the word for birthmark is *muttermal*, which means "mother's mark." In French, the word is *envie*, meaning a desire, and in Italian, the word is *voglia*, which means a wish or craving. Thus, it was believed that a pregnant woman's desire or craving for strawberries, for example, was responsible for a strawberry-colored mark on her unborn baby.

"Because vascular birthmarks are often found on the face and scalp, it was believed that women touched those same areas on themselves when frightened," says Dr. Mulliken. "Claret or port-wine stains were attributed to conception having taken place during menstruation."

Dr. Mulliken describes one of the most amusing examples of maternal imprinting. During the 18th century, a French woman gave birth to a baby whose birthmark so closely resembled the Phrygian cap — picture the soft blue hat worn by Smurfs — that the French government gave the mother 400 francs a year as an award for her patriotic thoughts!

IF YOU DECONSTRUCT A FACE, going deep below the epidermis, dermis, subcutaneous tissue, connective tissue, muscle, and bone, what do you have? "There is a set of assumptions based on how you look," says Case Western Reserve University's Dr. Hans. For example, if you're facially disfigured, others may assume you have mental deficits. If you're simply unattractive, the assumption may be that you've been blessed with intellect. If you're very attractive, people might assume you're an "airhead." There's a "brains line" and a "looks line." The assumption is that most people possess one or the other, but often not both.

We also make assumptions based on expressions. Humans have the most highly developed facial expressions in the animal world. Our expressions help us communicate emotions ranging from obvious, full-face feelings like surprise to subtle, fleeting displays of feeling like annoyance, all without the benefit of verbal communication. We depend on this nonverbal communication, which includes body language, as a way of getting our messages across clearly.

But if we don't look beyond the surface, we fail to consider the true person who lives inside each of us. Although the face is a portal for emotion and often gives clues about someone's personality and mood, it doesn't give away the entire secret. One man's kindness may not be reflected in his somber face, just as a woman's propensity for mean-spiritedness may be overlooked if she wears a broad smile.

For people with facial differences, the disparity is even more dramatic. They may appear to be grimacing when they are not, for example.

If their facial muscles don't function because of Moebius syndrome, or if they have severe scarring from a burn, they are unable to offer visual feedback during a conversation. Instead, they try to convey their emotions by their choice of words and tone of voice.

Look beyond the surface, because if you take someone at face value, you might as well judge a book by its cover.

❊

CHAPTER 3

where thou leadest me

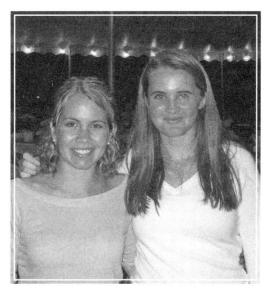

Nicole Reilly (right) and her friend Amy Mahon

I wake to sleep, and take my waking slow.
I feel my fate in what I cannot fear.
I learn by going where I have to go.

—Theodore Roethke, "The Waking"

DRIVING HOME WITH A bagel in her lap and sipping a cup of hot chocolate, Nicole Reilly was thinking that it was a perfect day to ski. The sky was clear, and the temperature wasn't too cold, considering that it was mid-February — Valentine's Day, actually. She was on her way home from a friend's house. They'd gone out together the night before to have a few drinks. Conscientious about not driving after drinking, Nicole spent the night at her friend's place.

She'd moved to Utah just a month earlier from New York, where her family still lived. During the day, she gave ski lessons at The Canyons, a ski resort in Park City — a ski scene from the James Bond movie *For Your Eyes Only* had been filmed there. At night, she worked as a bartender. Although she didn't have to work that day, she drove to the resort to test a new pair of skis. They were the "skis of the year," says Nicole, new high-end skis she'd heard great things about from her co-workers. She geared up and headed out. The day was perfect.

She skied for a few hours, thinking that she really liked the new skis. She decided to buy them. To get back to the base of the mountain, Nicole skied a back trail that wound around the middle of the mountain like a garland. With few other skiers on the trail, the skiing was peaceful and refreshing. Glints of ice, reflecting the noonday sun, appeared to dance across the landscape. Off the trail, the heavy snow looked like fondant icing on a birthday cake; the trees, like primitive candles.

"There was good snow coverage on the slope, but no moguls," says Nicole, referring to built-up snow resulting from the wind or created by skiers carving turns in the snow. The slope on the back trail was advanced, but it wasn't the "outer limits," she says, which are unmarked trails that sometimes offer skiers unwelcome surprises.

Wondering how much time she had before she needed to leave for her night job, Nicole pulled off to the side of the trail to check her watch. She had to be at the restaurant by about 5:30 and needed time to buy the skis and shower before going to work. Nicole looked down at her watch.

When she looked up, her parents were standing over her. She greeted them with a "hello" and then passed out. Later, she would remember hearing a voice ask, "What's your name? Where are you?" She was able to say, "Nicole Reilly," but she had no idea where she was.

NEILL REILLY, NICOLE'S FATHER, was at home on Long Island when he received a phone call that made no sense. "I thought it was someone trying to solicit me," he says, recalling the telephone call from the hospital in Utah. The caller was attempting to connect Neill with the surgeon in the trauma unit, but without being able to give him much information simply kept asking him to hold the line. Finally, Neill and the surgeon were connected.

"Is your daughter Nicole Reilly?" the surgeon asked.

"Yes," said Neill.

"Is she allergic to anything?"

"Yes," he replied again, "but I don't know what."

The surgeon then explained that Nicole had sustained a severe head trauma. They needed to perform brain imaging studies immediately, but needed to know whether she was allergic to anything. Nicole's mother, Linda, worked at a hospital at the time, about a half-hour from their home. With some effort, Neill was able to get Linda and the surgeon on the telephone together so Linda could relay Nicole's medical information.

"Your daughter has had a severe head trauma, an incident while skiing. She has a subdural hematoma. Blood on the brain. We're suggesting that she have brain surgery," said the surgeon.

"Is there anything else we can do?" Neill asked.

"Nothing else except wait and see if she lives," was the reply.

NICOLE GRADUATED FROM Lafayette College in 2000 with a double major in history and art. Not sure what she wanted to do with her life, she picked up a part-time job at a local yacht club, watching kids between their sailing lessons, and worked in retail for a while. She helped out at an interior design firm, discovering that a corporate environment was not suited to her style. She traveled to Spain and Ireland, then spent a week and a half in Chicago, Seattle, and Vancouver with a friend.

Still unsure of what she wanted to do but knowing that she loved the outdoors, she decided to head west to Utah to ski. "I always had a goal of becoming a much better skier," she says, describing herself as a cautious, conservative skier. "I didn't like to feel out of control. I'd do really hard trails, but I wouldn't make a point of skiing fast."

Nicole grew up on skis, often vacationing in Utah and upper Vermont with her parents. Utah was like a second home. "I already had a favorite restaurant," she says. She had the freedom and time to go, and the experience would allow her to think about what she wanted to do with her life.

NEILL AND LINDA SECURED the last two seats out of JFK International Airport to Salt Lake City that evening. Neill drove 80 miles an hour from their home to the airport and parked the car in the lot at the gate. "You don't want to leave unattended cars at JFK for days," says Neill, so he called his sister and asked if she'd pick up their car. She agreed. While Linda took care of checking them in, Neill rushed to the gate to hold the plane. The doors to the ramp that led to the plane were closing. Neill quickly explained the situation to the flight attendants. They couldn't miss the last plane out; what if Nicole didn't make it through the night? She was their only daughter. If she was going to die, they should be with her.

"If this would have happened post–9/11, they would have shot me," he says. But this was February, and 9/11 was still seven months away. Still, the situation was tense. The flight attendants weren't happy, he says, but they were willing to listen and to wait for Linda.

Just before Neill and Linda boarded the plane, they received a message on their cell phone that the surgery to relieve the pressure on Nicole's brain had gone well. In the face of their daughter's life-threatening situation, that positive news would get them through the plane ride. Still, they had no idea what to expect when they touched down in Utah four hours later. They passed the time the way most parents in that situation would: crying and praying.

Just outside the University of Utah Hospital's neuro intensive care unit, or NICU, Neill and Linda saw parents sleeping everywhere. At that moment, they realized they'd become full-fledged members of a unique club. They would spend the next couple of weeks listening to other parents' stories of car accidents and paralysis, and learning who was doing better, who was doing worse, and who didn't make it through the night. Many parents later told Neill and Linda that their daughter was in terrible shape when she arrived at the hospital — one of the worst cases they'd ever seen. Some weren't hopeful. Recalling the conversations with other parents, the waiting, the uncertainty, and his many discussions with God (sometimes out loud, he admits), Neill describes the experience simply by saying, "You're in hell."

Hooked up to a variety of flashing, beeping gizmos, with wires and tubes everywhere, Nicole lay motionless in her hospital bed. A handwritten sign over her bed read "Warning: Left flap is missing." Was that a good thing or a bad thing? At that moment, the questions started percolating, but Neill and Linda would find there were few solid answers. By some miracle, Nicole opened her eyes and greeted her parents with a "hello." Then she passed out again.

The physician showed Neill and Linda the results of the brain imaging study. He pointed out the blood on Nicole's brain, which, he said, could cause her to die or lose brain capacity. Because the hospital handled so many ski injury victims, the trauma team was able to use a radical surgical approach to relieve pressure building on the brain. Rather than boring holes into the skull and draining the excess fluid, the trauma team removed one of the skull plates that cover the brain.

The physician explained it to Nicole's parents this way: In head trauma cases, the skull is a friend to the brain during the impact because it helps protect the brain from injury. However, right after impact, the brain begins to swell, and the skull becomes the enemy. A swollen brain has nowhere to go. Death is not unusual. In Nicole's case, the left parietal bone, which makes up half the ceiling and one side of the entire skull, was completely removed.

"Where did you put it?" Neill asked.

"Don't worry; it's in the refrigerator," said the surgeon.

That would be one of the few questions to which Neill and Linda would get an answer. To the other thousand questions they asked, the reply was usually, "We hate to tell you this, but we just don't know." This scenario is typical with brain injuries.

Sometimes Nicole would wake up at night and, not understanding where she was, tear at her tubing. The intensive care nurses told Neill and Linda that this was a good sign. It meant she wanted to live.

THE DAY AFTER NICOLE arrived at the hospital, the ski instructor who'd rescued Nicole came to visit her. He told Neill and Linda that he'd been skiing and found a pair of skis in the snow on the side of the trail. Noticing a group of skiers farther down the trail, he skied to them to ask whether they had seen anything unusual or whether the skis belonged to them. When they replied no, he trekked back up the trail and took a closer look around. Several yards to the right, he spotted a young woman off the trail, covered in blood, stumbling around in the trees.

Nicole was semiconscious. He immediately checked her pulse. It was low, but it was on the radar. He sent his ski student down the hill to alert the ski patrol, which coordinated the rescue on the mountain. Once the paramedics got Nicole off the mountain, they headed for the University of Utah Hospital in Salt Lake City, where the staff specializes in head trauma. Even by ambulance, the trip took 45 minutes.

That Nicole was found so quickly after the accident, that the rescue was well coordinated, that she had access to experts in brain trauma, and that her brain hadn't yet swelled beyond recovery are what her father calls miracles. "The odds were insane," Neill says. "In essence, it was a relay race. If anyone had dropped the baton, Nicole would be dead or incapacitated. She is just off-the-charts lucky."

Triaging the acute frontotemporal subdural hematoma — Nicole's brain injury — was the trauma team's first priority. Secondary were the serious facial injuries that Nicole sustained, leaving her face terribly battered and bruised. She suffered fractures of the frontal sinus, left orbital area, and left zygomatic arch, which is part of the cheekbone that reaches to the front of the ear. Her zygomatic arch buckled outward as a result of her cheekbone being smashed in, and her left eye was pushed back into the socket. Amazingly, Nicole's injuries were totally limited to her face and head; nary a bruise or cut could be found anywhere on her body.

"We had to make some priorities," says Linda. After Nicole was treated for the traumatic brain injury, the next priority was to take care of the eye itself. Then they would treat her sinus fracture and, finally, repair the orbital area.

A week after her first surgery to relieve the pressure within her skull, known as intracranial pressure or ICP, Nicole underwent a second procedure to replace her skull plate, repair the frontal sinus fracture, and attempt an orbital reconstruction. One of her cranial nerves was entangled on a piece of fractured bone. As a result, Nicole's left pupil dilated dramatically, filling her iris completely, so that it appeared as though she had one blue eye and one black eye. The surgeons removed the impacted area around the nerve and began a repair of the fractures around her eye socket and cheekbone.

Nicole's parents met her in the recovery room following surgery. The surgery went well, and Nicole was in stable condition. So far, she had exceeded everyone's highest expectations. This second surgery was performed earlier than anticipated because she was doing so well.

"Everybody was in a good mood," recalls Linda. "She seemed to be on the road to recovery." Just to be sure, Neill asked the surgeon whether they needed to worry about Nicole dying. "You don't have to worry about her dying," said the surgeon.

Neill and Linda were at Nicole's bedside in the recovery room when, in the blink of an eye, she began trembling. Something wasn't right. Her skull plate had been removed during the first operation to relieve the growing pressure inside her head. But after surgeons replaced the plate, her brain began to swell again, and her intracranial pressure began to build rapidly. If not relieved quickly, Nicole would suffer brain damage or even die. Neill raced down the hall and found an orderly, who ran back to Nicole's room, with other staff following on his heels. By this time, Nicole's heart rate, which ordinarily is 45, was over 180.

"Oh my God, she's going under!" cried the orderly.

"Come back!" cried her mother.

"I can't do it anymore," whispered Nicole from beneath her bandages. "I'm not staying."

Neill and Linda watched as their only daughter was rushed away on a gurney. The surgeon's words, "You don't have to worry about her dying," seemed like a curse.

The staff packed Nicole in ice to induce hypothermia quickly, which would reduce the swelling of her brain. To gauge her level of consciousness, they took turns pinching and slapping her arms — standard practice, as odd as it may seem. To relieve the pressure inside Nicole's head, an intracranial pressure bolt was drilled into her forehead. The tip of the bolt was inserted into the cerebrospinal fluid–filled ventricle inside her brain. Called a ventriculostomy, the procedure allows the cerebrospinal fluid to drain, relieving the intracranial pressure and preventing brain damage or death.

The next day, Nicole still wasn't in great shape, but she was coherent enough to impart words of caution to her mother. "Don't let them bring me to the basement," she said. "They slap you down there."

Her intracranial pressure finally stabilized, and Nicole essentially fell asleep for a week. Then, just two weeks after she'd arrived at the University of Utah Hospital and to the surprise of her parents, her physician released her. Only later would Nicole learn how uncertain her prognosis had been.

NICOLE ARRIVED HOME from the hospital on March 1, 2001. Back at home, she obsessed about the accident. She would make her way down to the breakfast table each morning and quiz her parents. "What happened to me?" she'd ask, and then, "Why did this happen?" Every day, seven days a week, month after month, she'd ask the same questions over and over.

The answer to the first question was always the same. No one really knew what had happened. The most plausible theory was that another skier had been flying down the slope and come up behind Nicole — even though she had stopped along the side of the trail — hitting her with such tremendous force that she was cast into the air and then violently thrown to the ground. She never saw a thing. She's left-handed and wears her watch on her right hand. When she pulled over to the side of the trail to check the time, her head was turned to the right. She would not have seen anyone coming from the left, down the slope.

This dark void in the story was terribly frustrating. One moment, Nicole was standing in the middle of a snow-covered mountain, engaged in a minute detail of everyday life. She blinked and ended up in a hospital bed. Those were the facts she could hold in her hands, and no amount of asking "What happened to me?" would shed any new details. Chances are, that piece of the story is lost forever — tucked away deep inside the conscience of someone who will never come forward, never say "I'm sorry," never explain what happened and why he or she didn't stop. For now, Nicole's is a story with a severed plot, an unknown antagonist, and an imprecise ending.

The answer to why it happened was much more difficult, although Neill understood Nicole's relentless obsession with wanting an answer. "It's human nature to delve into your own personal tragedy, like a hamster in a wheel, going around and around and around," he says.

Still, the exercise was frustrating for everyone. Linda says she spent hours and hours holding Nicole's hand while she would ask the question over and over again. "It was a sad kind of rumination," she recalls. Any answer her parents offered Nicole wasn't easily received. Linda would tell her that sometimes things happen to allow us to appreciate what we have, and Nicole would counter emphatically, "But I loved my life. I didn't disregard my life."

So Linda would tell her that perhaps that very question is the meaning. She'd say, "It's enough to have the question, because the question is going to make you proceed a little further and in the end provide wisdom for you."

SOMETIME IN MAY, about three months after the accident, the swelling in Nicole's face finally subsided, and the true extent of her facial injuries appeared. Linda recalls looking at Nicole and thinking, "Oh my, my. There's a problem."

Nicole expected the surgeries performed at the University of Utah Hospital to be the only ones she'd need. "I wasn't really with it, so I wasn't thinking about the outcome," she says. She had no expectations because no one explained the extent of her facial injuries or even let her see her face until the end of her second week in the hospital. Even so, most of her visible injuries were masked by the ferocious swelling.

Nicole's facial injuries were concentrated in the area of her left eye, which had sunk deep into her face. Her left upper lid hung down, giving her eye a half-closed look. The area from her eyebrow to her cheekbone sloped downward and inward, while the bone from her ear to the edge of her eye — the zygomatic arch — bowed outward, causing that side of her face to appear especially wide and uneven compared with the right side. From Nicole's perspective, the insult to her injury was the fact that her entire head had been shaved in order to perform the cranial surgery.

"The one side of her face was very different from the other side," says Linda, adding that the human brain expects symmetry in a face and can tolerate only a slight variation. "It was devastating every time she looked in the mirror."

Nicole consulted an otolaryngologist (ear, nose, and throat doctor) on Long Island, who said her sinus repair looked perfect. "You won't ever have a problem with it," she told Nicole, who then asked the physician about fixing her eye. She informed Nicole that she was missing volume in the eye and said, "I don't touch that."

Nicole's parents turned to *New York Magazine*, which publishes an annual list of the top doctors in the area. Through the list, they found several ophthalmologists, all of whom met with Nicole and her parents. Each doctor told them something different, leaving them confused and unsure of what to do.

One ophthalmologist advised Nicole to buy a pair of glasses with a magnification of .2 on the left and no magnification on the right. This way, the eye would appear normal when Nicole looked at someone. That she would probably fall down a flight of stairs because she was wearing a wrong prescription lens seemed secondary. Another said he wouldn't attempt a repair for fear of damaging her remaining eyesight. Still another said he couldn't help, but he did tell them to make sure no one touched her good eye, no matter what, in an attempt to create symmetry. Nicole and her parents had gotten no further than when they began. No one would help.

TOWARD THE END OF MAY, after being home from the hospital just three months, Nicole signed up for two classes, psychology and ceramics, at Nassau Community College. She felt she'd recuperated long enough. "I think I was trying to find a way to get my life back. I felt that I had to get out and live," she says. Getting back into school would get Nicole out of the house, test her ability to sit in a classroom, and keep her education on track.

Although Nicole progressed beautifully from her brain injury, the other losses resulting from the accident were difficult for her to comprehend. Suddenly Nicole's familiar, comfortable life stopped and she was forced to acknowledge these strangers at the door. Minor cognitive issues demanded attention. She was lagging behind her friends, who were either in school or beginning careers. Her own image was a stranger, the face in the mirror so different from the one she had known before.

Says Linda, "Her constant statement was 'You know, I can't under-stand this happening at my age. I just didn't expect this.'" Every loss is painful, but mysterious losses, like that of a family member who doesn't show up for breakfast one morning and whose well-worn slippers sit beside the side door, wrap themselves around us, feeding us endless loops of questions that keep us from grieving and thus healing.

AT THE END OF AUGUST, Nicole and her parents found an ophthal-mologist who was willing to try to correct the positioning of Nicole's eye. The ophthalmologist performed two procedures on Nicole, one in October and another in February 2002, but he wasn't concerned about the related cosmetic issues and reluctantly referred them to a facial reconstructive surgeon at New York University Medical Center.

All of Nicole's X-rays and records were sent to the facial reconstruc-tive surgeon for his review. Eight weeks passed without hearing a word from the surgeon. Finally, Linda called the doctor's office and asked whether the surgeon could help Nicole, "because if not, we have to find someone." The next day, Linda received a call from the surgeon's office. The message was that he never operates on a site where someone else has been.

"We were at a dead end," says Linda.

Then one evening, Neill and Linda were watching CNN's *Larry King Live*. Louise Ashby, an aspiring actress who was badly injured in a car accident in Los Angeles in 1992, was Larry's guest. Nicole's par-ents called her into the living room to watch with them. Louise had undergone significant facial reconstruction (she has 238 metal plates in her skull) by one of the nation's top reconstructive surgeons, Dr. Henry Kawamoto Jr.

Nicole and her parents had an idea. They had been planning a visit to Los Angeles to visit a relative. Why not combine the trip with an appointment with Dr. Kawamoto? The next day, Nicole called Dr. Kawamoto's office and told the receptionist her story. When she said she'd be coming in from New York, the receptionist asked, "Why don't you call Dr. Kawamoto's former craniofacial fellow, David Staffenberg? He's in the Bronx." Eureka!

That it took Nicole and her parents months and months of effort to find a physician to help them didn't surprise Dr. Staffenberg, who is chief of Pediatric Plastic Surgery and the director of Craniofacial Surgery at the Children's Hospital at Montefiore in New York City. Too often, he says, "patients are not sure of the road map — who can help them or where they should go for what kind of surgery."

When Nicole met with Dr. Staffenberg, she found him kind and honest. "He said, 'You know, Nicole, this is going to be a very tough case. It depends on how far you can stick with this and keep your spirits up and work with me.' He was willing to stick with me until I felt secure about how I look."

Dr. Staffenberg outlined the issues he found along the left side of Nicole's face: Her eye was sunken, her eyebrow sagging; the zygomatic arch was not right, and until the bone was fixed, it didn't matter what was done around the eye. Everyone else had thought that if the eyebrow was raised and the eye pulled forward, Nicole's face would be fine. The heart of the problem, as Dr. Staffenberg saw it, was that Nicole's cheekbone was "pushed straight back into her face" and the zygomatic arch was pushed out. As he saw it, once her cheek was repaired, the eye could be tackled.

"All of these seemingly separate elements actually work together," he says.

Not until then did Nicole and her parents really understand how all the injuries related to one another. Nicole's face no longer comprised separate parts that required attention from multiple unknown specialists, working independently from one another. Her face was the sum of its parts, and one person, who understood and shared the family's goals and concerns, could help put the pieces back together in a logical, meaningful way.

The first step that Dr. Staffenberg proposed was to remove the metal plates and screws that held Nicole's cheekbone in its incorrect position and then re-create the fractures, using a small electric saw. The cheekbone could then be repositioned and secured. While he described this as the best approach, Nicole and her parents favored an alternative, more conservative approach, whereby the bone beneath her eye that had been smashed in would be built up. To accomplish that, Dr. Staffenberg would need extra bone, either from Nicole's body or a cadaver, or artificial material.

A patient's own tissue is always preferred because it offers a lower risk of rejection and infection than cadaveric bone or artificial implants do, even despite recent advances. For example, some physicians are using an investigational technique in which cadaveric bone and artificial implants are combined with molecular growth factors to aid in healing. Dr. Staffenberg, however, is cautious. "It's a tremendous advance, but we still don't know what those medications will do years down the road," he says, adding that they may encourage more rapid healing, or they may fail or perhaps even encourage tumor growth. "When most patients are infants and children and young adults, we can't help but have those worries."

Current artificial materials sometimes cause chronic problems with infections or act like deeply embedded splinters, somehow finding their way out, he explains. Chin implants, for example, can work their way out or can move inward and embed in the roots of the lower teeth. Patients who have a chin implant should understand the risks. This way, if they have a problem with their lower teeth, they'll know it might be related to the implant and know what to ask their physician, says Dr. Staffenberg.

"To avoid that kind of problem in someone who is young like Nicole, we want to use something that has the best chance of healing and being permanent," he says. "When someone like Nicole comes along, you can imagine we frequently say, 'Although it may be easy for us to take something artificial out of a package, we know what some of the risks might be.' We know how to use the patient's own bone and how to obtain it. We still have to consider this the gold standard. If there's a reason we couldn't use the patient's own tissue, then we consider using artificial or cadaveric tissue."

In Nicole's case, he chose to take bone from the top of her skull, employing a procedure called a split calvarial bone graft. Nicole recalls Dr. Staffenberg describing skull bone as being ideally suited for repairing delicate areas of the body, such as the face. Dr. Staffenberg explains that the skull is composed of three layers. The outer layer, which is solid bone, can be taken as graft material. The thin middle layer, which is soft and spongy, and the inner layer stay intact to protect the brain.

Although the patient's own tissue is the "gold standard," getting the donor bone or tissue is often the difficult part of the surgery, as well as the most painful for the patient. For example, performing a split calvarial bone graft is delicate, precise work, done with drills and fine chisels, explains Dr. Staffenberg. The trick is to remove the bone from the top of the skull without injuring the brain or fracturing the skull.

After Dr. Staffenberg performed the split calvarial bone graft, he shaped the outer layer of bone and placed it on the cheek, securing it with screws. In time, the new bone would integrate with the rest of the facial bones. Finally, he shaved down Nicole's zygomatic arch to minimize its outward bowing and to help restore symmetry to her face.

Next, Dr. Staffenberg could attend to her eye. The fractures around Nicole's eye socket were like fault lines, weakening the entire area. Because the floor of her eye socket was shattered, it collapsed downward, causing her eyeball to sink into her skull. Her eye fell inward roughly eight millimeters, which is about a third of an inch. Dr. Staffenberg brought her left eye forward by building up the bone in her socket behind the eyeball — again using bone from Nicole's skull.

"Being able to move the eye forward after that kind of injury, among surgeons, is considered to be a very difficult thing," says Dr. Staffenberg. One danger is that the optic nerve will be damaged or the blood supply to the nerve will be affected if the eye is moved forward after it already has undergone some healing. In fact, it's possible to be blinded by this surgery, he says. To prevent further injury to Nicole's eye, he moved her eye forward in stages. He would move her eye forward a few millimeters, allow it to heal, and allow the blood supply to adapt.

"Sometimes, you can't do something in one fell swoop and expect a good outcome," he says.

In less than three years, Dr. Staffenberg has performed six reconstructive surgeries on Nicole, each one progressing closer to the final goal. The last few procedures were done to adjust the position of the eyelid and the outer corner of the eye, and to try to improve the symmetry that she lost. Nicole also has undergone procedures to correct entropion, which is an inward rolling of the eyelid that is quite painful because the eyelashes continually scratch the eye. Dr. Staffenberg also added more bone to the eye socket to bring her left eye out farther.

All of her facial reconstruction was done in a manner that minimized scarring. Surgeons can enter the face from inside the mouth (underneath the lip in front of the teeth, for example), from behind the eyelid, through the pink part behind the eyelashes, or through the forehead above the ear, Dr. Staffenberg explains. "It's a sneaky way of getting in there without leaving scars."

To this day, Nicole and her parents wonder why no one — not the highly regarded eye surgeons, brain surgeons, ophthalmologists, or other physicians they'd seen — referred them to a craniofacial team. Nicole could have gotten help sooner and perhaps even avoided some surgeries. For example, to correct her ptosis, which is sagging of the upper eyelid, her eyelid was shortened. The shortened eyelid better fit her eye, but the eye was still sunken. Subsequently, when her eye was brought forward, she didn't have enough eyelid for the procedure, so Dr. Staffenberg had to reconstruct that, too.

"She's had so many surgeries and some of them she probably didn't even need," says Linda. "We had no game plan and didn't know where to turn."

BETWEEN SURGERIES, NICOLE worked some part-time jobs, one of which was at a doctor's office. "They thought I should pick up some science classes and go to medical school," says Nicole. She decided that perhaps that was the meaning behind her accident: She was meant to become a great doctor. She applied to Columbia University and was accepted.

In May 2003, Dr. Staffenberg performed a procedure to push out Nicole's eye 12 millimeters. The procedure caused double vision that lasted for months. By that time, Nicole was at the end of her first semester of her second year at Columbia and was struggling. The constant double vision was a huge barrier to learning and studying, not to mention simply living her life.

"I had to figure out where to sit because the professor had two heads," she says.

The entropion came back, and no matter how many eyedrops she used, her eyelashes constantly scratched her eye. She had to drop out of school. "I was way too far behind, way too defeated. That put an end to my idea of medical school."

Nicole felt stranded. She took many steps forward, but never seemed to get closer to a goal. "People in their twenties have a hard enough time. It doesn't help to have something this strange happen to me," she says. "I graduated from school, and my friends were moving forward with their lives. I was stuck at square one." Nicole began ruminating again about why the accident happened, the question burning a hole in her tender psyche.

The desire for absolutes, for answers to the question "Why did this happen?" is rooted in our existential mind. From understanding and explaining the meaning of our existence to knowing the reason that a particular event occurred, we crave order, logic, and meaning. Random events are unsettling. Did that car pull out in front of me today because I needed to slow down and appreciate my life or because, in an act of haste that was sure to turn the world upside down, I moved my good luck charm from my rearview mirror to my coat pocket? We simply don't accept random events easily.

Because Nicole's injury so profoundly affected her physically, mentally, socially, and academically, she believed there had to be a reason it happened. It simply couldn't have been a case of bad luck or "accidents happen." Eventually, she stopped asking "Why me?" and began thinking, "Okay, it was me. What am I supposed to do now? What am I supposed to learn from this?" Somewhere tucked inside her experience, she believed there was a higher purpose.

Had she found great happiness, great fortune in Utah, would she have asked the same questions? Would any of us? We may be thankful when our lives are happy and carefree, but we seldom ask why we are so lucky or wonder about the meaning behind our good fortune. We may feel optimistic or grumble anyway for dramatic effect, but we keep going on our way. For some reason, most of us search for meaning only from pain. Are our losses any more meaningful than our happiness and good fortune?

Each of Nicole's family members has struggled to find meaning in her experience. A strong Irish Catholic family, the Reillys, particularly Neill, looked to their faith for answers to Nicole's questions. "Somehow in the secret of Christianity is this mystery of pain, suffering, and redemption," says Neill. "Somehow pain and suffering have meaning, and that is really hard to accept, but it's better than pain having no meaning."

Many evenings were filled with conversation about the ultimate sacrifice in Christianity—Jesus dying on the cross—and its meaning: that all people would be saved, their pain and suffering reduced. Neill says that, like Christ, people who have really hard lives are heroic because they've taken on more pain and suffering than others, which reduces the pain and suffering for the rest of us. Somewhere along the way, on a deeply spiritual level, perhaps, Nicole's father thinks she may have made the choice to accept an extra share of pain.

The second time Nicole almost died was the most trying for Neill. He stood on the edge of hell, shouting upward to the heavens: "This is stupid, God! Why would you let her go through this just to let her die! She's been through so much! Why let her survive just to go through more pain and then die?" He bargained with God to let Nicole live, he says, giving God his best sales pitch ever.

Through her conversations with her parents and her own reflection and prayer, Nicole has determined that suffering makes people stronger, allowing them to help others. "While on Earth, people are tested, and their ability to persevere through trying times enables them to become stronger," she says.

IN JULY 2005, DR. STAFFENBERG performed another reconstructive surgery on Nicole. He lifted her left eyebrow, opened the outside corner of her eye, treated the entropion, and pushed her eye out another one to two millimeters. He shaved down her zygomatic arch and lifted her cheek. Just about a year later, he performed more work to further correct her zygomatic arch.

"Part of the obligation of the surgeon before doing any kind of reconstruction like this is making sure the patients have a really good understanding of not just the surgical risks and benefits, but also an idea of what realistic expectation there can be as each step is taken," he says, adding that Nicole understands how complicated reconstruction can be.

"A human face is different from the body of a car," says Dr. Staffenberg. "It's living tissue, and manipulating living tissue is so much more difficult." He notes that one cannot always predict the way tissue will heal. For instance, the entropion, the lower eyelid rolling back into the eye, has since returned.

"He was very honest from the get-go," says Nicole. "He said, 'You'll never be restored one hundred percent.'" And then she says something that perhaps only people with ongoing medical problems can truly understand: "I want there to be an end, but I don't want there to be an end."

NICOLE'S MOTHER HAS STRUGGLED with the question of how much surgery is enough surgery. "Each new surgery is fraught with anxiety.

Is she going to be okay? Are our standards too high? Is there anything more to be gained?" Linda says. Yet she knows how primary appearance is to each of us and how Nicole's facial injuries affected her sense of self.

"It impacts everything," says Linda. "It's impacted her self-esteem, social sense, relationship with friends. It's impacted her ability to really put herself out there. I'm talking about someone who was really socially outgoing. She was the social secretary in her sorority in college." The change in Nicole, says Linda, was a real U-turn.

Nicole says she hasn't dated since the accident five years ago. "Now, I think it would be nice, but I feel anxious and uncomfortable," she says, wondering how people perceive her. Do they see her as she sees herself: crooked, misshapen?

"It's probably much worse in my own mind," says Nicole. "I'm working on being more confident," noting that at least her face is improved and her hair has grown back to the length it was before the accident. Still, she says, "Sometimes I look in the mirror and I don't recognize myself. I think I'm silly and too critical, but at the same time because it's me, I can't escape that."

"The ego resides in the body, and when you have such an insult to your ego, to reclaim that territory takes a lot of struggle," says Linda. Particularly when you're young and insecure anyway, looking different from everyone else affects how you relate to others, and that affects all aspects of your life. "Like a house of cards," Linda says.

WHEN NICOLE LEFT FOR Utah a handful of years ago, she had no idea where her life was going to take her. At 28, she was back in school full time, with plans to get her BSN/master's degree in nursing and thinking about specializing in pediatrics, especially treating children with special needs.

"I don't think any of that would have happened if it weren't for the accident," says Linda. "I believe she'll be able to help a lot of people."

Nicole thinks less often now about the accident and why it happened, although she is reminded every time she looks in a mirror. "The way I see it, I'm always going to have to work on accepting it," she says.

She volunteered for several months in the Child Life Department at North Shore University Hospital to get a feel for the hospital environment. Once, she played checkers with a boy of about ten who was a patient in the pediatric intensive care unit. His body was tethered to a bundle of machines. Game after game, he beat Nicole, giggling through his oxygen mask and thinking it quite curious that she had forgotten how to play. She was struck by his lighthearted nature, despite his serious health problems.

She says, "He made me realize that I really can't let myself get that upset about things."

CHAPTER 4

the gunner with the silver mask

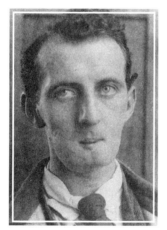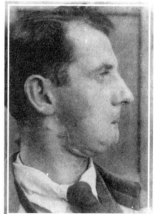

Corporal Fred Snowden

The head injuries were the most frightful, for in some cases
the greater part of the face was smashed in by shrapnel, while in
others the nose, eye, and greater part of the cheek had been
torn away, leaving a great, red, bleeding cavity.

> —Dr. William Boyd, 3rd Canadian
> Field Ambulance, Battle of Neuve
> Chapelle, March 13, 1915

DURING THE SIEGE OF Antwerp in 1832, Monsieur Alphonse Louis, a 22-year-old French artillery gunner, was severely injured by a large piece of shrapnel from an exploding shell. The shrapnel ripped apart his left cheek, destroyed his soft palate, and tore off most of his lower jaw. Ordinarily, an injury like this would have been fatal; in this case, M. Louis survived because of rapid rescue efforts and excellent field care.

One year later, Sir William Whymper of the Grenadier Guards recalled the event in an article published in the *London Medical Gazette*. He described the extensive tissue loss in M. Louis's face, noting in detail how the bottom of his tongue had been sliced away, all the way to the throat. Without a lower jaw or its usual tissue and muscle support, the tongue simply hung out of what was left of M. Louis's mouth.

Whymper wrote that, despite the quick evacuation to the military field hospital, it was felt that M. Louis would not survive long. Surely, his case was among the most tragic that army surgeons had encountered: His injuries were horrific, and yet he was still alive. He underwent surgery to stop the bleeding from his facial injuries, and his right forearm, which had been hit by shrapnel, was amputated about two inches below the elbow.

According to Whymper's account, roughly a week and a half passed before his doctor felt that M. Louis might actually survive. He suffered terribly, and his wounds became infected and gangrenous. Still, he was given "the most energetic treatment" and "the most indefatigable attention," both of which surely contributed to his survival.

Because of his missing lower jaw, M. Louis was unable to eat or speak well. He was sustained by a diet of watery broth, eventually graduating to more solid, albeit soft, foods, all of which were slipped directly down his throat. His appearance also was hugely affected. In his account, Whymper notes that M. Louis's tongue drooped and he "dribbled saliva constantly." Although the army surgeon saved his life, physicians at that time didn't have the expertise to rebuild destroyed faces. But necessity is the mother of invention, and M. Louis surely needed a lower jaw. Thus, it was decided that a mask, uniquely fabricated by a silversmith, might do the trick.

After many weeks, the injuries to M. Louis's face were healed enough so that a plaster cast could be taken of his face. His surgeon oversaw the functional design. The silversmith, an artist in Antwerp named Jan Pieter Antoon Verschuylen, used the cast to fashion a mask of silver, which he painted with flesh-colored oils to match the rest of the face. Whiskers and a mustache were added to make the mask appear more lifelike. When it was finished, the mask weighed three pounds.

Although one might think the mask was nothing more than a fancy cover-up for M. Louis's severe facial injuries, that was not at all the case. The mask, which was affixed to his head with straps, was equipped with a hinge and spring that allowed him to open and close his new jaw. Whymper noted in his article that the mask not only was functional (the ingenious design actually allowed M. Louis to eat and speak), but also allowed him to live a relatively normal life. He wrote:

> On our last visit to Alphonse Louis, the day previous to his departure for Lille, he appeared in high spirits; he walked about with agility; used the stump of the forearm with address; took off and readjusted his mask with his left hand; spoke not only intelligibly but easily; he was high coloured and fatter, as he stated, than he had ever been prior to his misfortune. He played at cards, and seemed to be as proud of shewing [showing] the mechanisms of his artificial jaw, as he was of the crosses of the Legion of Honour and Leopold, that glittered on his bosom.

After Whymper's last visit to M. Louis, we do not know what became of the soldier, whose bravery and will to survive are reflected in his legendary nickname, "The Gunner with the Silver Mask." We only can hope that he lived out the rest of his days comfortably, thanks to the perseverance and skill of a surgeon and an artist, as well as a good bit of luck.

ROUGHLY 100 YEARS LATER, the "Great War" or the "War to End All Wars," as World War I was called, broke out. Unlike the wars and battles before it, World War I would change the face of wartime injuries dramatically.

Before World War I, soldiers were largely mobile. Enemies would converge at a remote location to settle their differences, far from towns or villages pulsing with innocent civilians, women, and children. Situated on the battlefield, the soldiers would advance, fight, and retreat or advance further, depending on whose army was mightier. At battle's end, the wounded and dead were collected, and they called it a day. At that time, war was almost gentlemanly.

During World War I, a new style of fighting and new methods of killing and maiming were introduced. Trench warfare turned formerly mobile men into sitting ducks. The men dug rows of trenches in the earth, large enough for them to live inside, and there they stayed. The soldiers slept and ate in the muddy and often water-filled trenches. They fought vermin, disease, and the enemy in the trenches. They composed songs, told jokes, cried, and died in the trenches.

Unlike the weapons of earlier wars, the weapons of choice during World War I had incredible killing range. They could be launched from a great distance, minimizing close-range warfare and hand-to-hand combat but increasing the physical devastation. Artillery shells, machine guns, hand grenades, and bombs were added to the armament of rifles, bayonets, and cannons.

Beyond the trenches was the place where the enemy and danger lurked, the place called "no-man's-land." Invariably a soldier would feel the need to poke his head out of the trench and gaze toward that mysterious place. If the enemy's artillery shells missed him, its snipers took a chance. Despite the protection offered by steel helmets, many soldiers sustained horrific injuries to their faces and heads, giving surgeons plenty of opportunity to pioneer medical advances to treat devastating facial injuries.

Sir Harold Gillies was one such surgeon and is considered by many to be the father of plastic and reconstructive surgery. Originally from New Zealand, he was trained as an otolaryngologist.

Rather than wait to be drafted, Dr. Gillies joined the Red Cross when the war broke out. Dr. Andrew Bamji, curator of the Gillies Archives at Queen Mary's Hospital, Sidcup, in England, says that Dr. Gillies assisted a dentist named Auguste Valadier in Wimereux, outside Boulogne, who was doing some facial work at the 83rd General Hospital. Dr. Valadier specialized in treating injuries to the jaw and was experimenting with tissue grafting, a concept that fascinated Dr. Gillies.

"Valadier had no medical qualifications, so he was not allowed to operate unsupervised," says Dr. Bamji. Thus, Dr. Gillies took advantage of the opportunity to assist and learn from Dr. Valadier.

In Paris, Dr. Gillies observed Hippolyte Morestin, a well-respected plastic surgeon who treated patients using flap surgery, a technique dating back to ancient India and one that is still used today.

FLAP SURGERY INVOLVES transferring flaps of skin and tissue from healthy parts of the body to the wound site. As far as anyone can tell, sometime between 600 B.C. and the first century A.D., an Indian surgeon named Sushruta recorded the method of rebuilding a nose using what's called a pedicle flap. According to records, the wound was "anointed with honey and clarified butter," covered with "cotton and linen, and tied with strings of thread," and then finally dusted with baked clay powders.

In ancient India, the face — the nose, in particular — was a common target of violence. In fact, rhinokopia, or nose disfigurement, was an accepted form of punishment for all types of crimes, including adultery. Perhaps because it emerges so proudly from the center of the face, the nose is the seat of honor and leadership. Having one's nose destroyed was tremendously humiliating, and hiding the damage was not easily accomplished — yet another incentive for the enemy.

The practice of targeting the nose as a punishment extended beyond India. During the Byzantine era, rhinokopia was performed to prevent a man from ascending the throne. According to Byzantine law, an emperor could not have an obvious physical deformity; thus, a man without a nose clearly could not rule.

Byzantine emperor Justinian II was known as Rhinotmetus, or the "one with an amputated nose," after he was overthrown and his nose mutilated to prevent him from regaining power. Whether he was fitted with a prosthetic nose or underwent nasal reconstruction is a matter of some debate. In any event, Justinian II did return to power following some type of nasal repair, but was later overthrown and beheaded — an insult no surgeon could hope to correct.

Pedicle flap surgery in India was an amazing innovation for its time. Called the "Indian" or "Hindu" method, the technique involved matching a plant leaf to the area of skin to be replaced. The surgeon would then place the leaf on the patient's forehead or, more likely, the cheek. Next, much as one would use a stencil, the surgeon would cut out a piece of skin the same size as the leaf, leaving one edge of skin attached. This way, the tissue to be transferred still had an adequate blood supply that would nourish the tissue's regrowth. The wound site was then scarified, or "freshened" as it were, to allow the flap to be attached. Once healed, the connection was cut and any excess skin removed. This technique was not documented in Europe until roughly the 15th century, when it was reintroduced by an Italian surgeon, Gaspare Tagliacozzi.

Like all medical procedures during that time, flap surgery was accomplished without the benefit of antibiotics or anesthesia. In fact, in an article published in the *Boston Medical and Surgical Journal* (now the *New England Journal of Medicine*) in 1837 describing the pedicle flap technique, the author notes the patient's tolerance of the procedure without anesthesia: "During the whole of this long and painful operation, the patient kept up his courage, and not a cry was uttered, nor the least struggle made that could at all impede the motions of the operator." Thankfully, by 1846, inhaled ether was introduced as a surgical anesthesia.

DR. GILLIES IMPROVED the pedicle flap technique, creating what he called the tubed pedicle graft. This innovation was as much the result of his keen mind as it was of his surgical skill. On an October evening in 1917, while Dr. Gillies was working at Queen Mary's Hospital in Sidcup, he was presented with a navy general named Yeo, whose face had been badly burned in an explosion on the HMS *Warspite* during the Battle of Jutland. Historical records show that the patient's eyelids and lower lip were turned inside out and his nose was burned nearly off.

Dr. Gillies fashioned a complete cover for General Yeo's nose and cheeks using skin from his chest, leaving one edge connected to ensure a blood supply. He cut a hole out of the skin for a mouth and stitched the flap into place. And then he realized something he'd never noticed before: When such a large flap of skin was cut away from its original site, it curled into a tube. He considered the potential: "If I stitched the edges of those flaps together, might I not create a tube of living tissue which would increase the blood supply to grafts, close them to infection, and be far less liable to contract or degenerate as the older methods were?" This innovation also would allow for a greater distance between the wound site and the donor site.

Thus, the tubed pedicle graft was born. Interestingly, the tubed pedicle graft also was pioneered about the same time by Russian surgeon Vladimir Petrovich Filatov. Surgeons around the world used the technique routinely until the 1970s.

Recognizing the advantages of flap surgery, Dr. Gillies used the technique not only to provide functional facial reconstruction but also to give his patients the most normal appearance possible. Unlike other surgeons of his day, he possessed an exquisite sense of aesthetics. A colleague of his once wrote, "In many hundreds of hours spent assisting or in watching Gillies in the operating room I never once saw him perform a hurried or rough movement. All the actions of his hands were consistently gentle, accurate and deft."

Another innovation resulted from Dr. Gillies caring for General Yeo, says Dr. Bamji. The burns around Yeo's eyes had contracted the skin, so he was unable to blink. An inability to blink can cause scarring of the cornea, because the eyes get dry. Gillies was bothered by this enough to pioneer a method of restoring function and appearance to his patient. The method became known as the epithelial outlay technique, and it was an immediate success.

Dr. Gillies described his work as "a strange new art," and he was the first surgeon to use drawings of his patients both before and after surgery to describe the reconstruction. An ex-surgeon and teacher at the Slade School of Art named Henry Tonks worked with him, eventually establishing a name for himself as a World War I graphic historian and artist.

Dr. Gillies's work, initially at Aldershot, outgrew its facilities with the start of the Battle of the Somme, and he was given the go-ahead to establish a hospital in Sidcup devoted exclusively to facial surgery. In 1920, he used his experience as the basis for a consummate reference guide to his specialty: *Plastic Surgery of the Face.*

"Up until Gillies, no single surgeon had accumulated either the experience or the team to do things on a grand scale," says Dr. Bamji. "Although many techniques had been described, the numbers of patients allowed them to be refined. His approach was systematic."

The epithelial outlay technique and tubed pedicle graft were not his only innovations. Later in his career, Dr. Gillies established a new principle in the treatment of nasal disfigurement from leprosy, using what he called an intranasal skin graft. He also pioneered a new method for reattaching severed limbs.

Between the two world wars, Dr. Gillies increasingly handled cosmetic cases. However, most of his patients were people seeking relief from facial injuries and disfigurement resulting from accidents, burns, congenital deformities, and tumors. He always considered cosmetic surgery to be nothing more than a "subordinate extension of reconstructive surgery."

ANOTHER PIONEER IN FACIAL reconstruction was Varaztad Kazanjian, known as the "Miracle Man of the Western Front." Native to Turkish Armenia, Dr. Kazanjian fled to America to escape the Armenian holocaust in 1895, becoming a U.S. citizen in 1900. When World War I broke out, the British desperately needed dental specialists, and Dr. Kazanjian, who trained as a dentist at Harvard Dental School, volunteered. He joined the first Harvard Unit, which was stationed in France.

He handled more than 3,000 cases of gunshot, shrapnel, and other wounds of the face and jaw, including the case of Lance Corporal Fred Snowden, who sustained a shell wound that ripped apart his mouth, chin, and lower face. Dr. Kazanjian operated on him, rebuilding his lower jaw and mouth. In a letter to Dr. Kazanjian in 1918, two years after his surgery, Snowden wrote: "It would take too long to go through all that has been said about my face by professional men — dozens have examined it + all agree…that it is a masterpiece."

After returning from the war, Dr. Kazanjian enrolled at Harvard Medical School. While in class one day, he was observing a surgical technique demonstrated by Dr. Harvey Cushing and two high-ranking officials from the Royal Army Medical Corps. The two officials recognized Dr. Kazanjian and pulled him from the audience, introducing him as the man who had first shown them the very technique they were about to demonstrate.

A humble and unassuming man, Dr. Kazanjian was acutely aware of the psychological effects of facial deformities and attempted to tailor treatments to the individual patients. In doing so, he pioneered some of his own innovations while serving in the army. For example, he pioneered the use of splints and wires to repair complex jaw injuries, once spending half a year crafting special dentures for a sailor who had lost his upper jaw. The design involved a series of rods and wires that connected to the upper part of the sailor's face. Dr. Kazanjian was pleased with the outcome, until Ripley sensationalized it with the headline "Believe it or not — Dr. Kazanjian made a man chew with his eyebrows!"

Although renowned, Dr. Kazanjian didn't take credit for his work, saying, "It was not I, nor was it my assistants. It was the great need of the time that evolved the technique which made it possible for injured men to speak again, to look something like they had before. Take the need, add patience and hope, and resourcefulness, and you have the ingredients that will bring the surgeon to success."

Several other plastic surgeons made tremendous contributions to healing those with facial disfigurement, among them Dr. John Peter Mettauer, who performed the nation's first cleft palate surgery in 1827, and Dr. Vilray Blair, who established a solid surgical infrastructure during World War I to accommodate the large number of men with head and neck injuries.

DESPITE THE MEDICAL ADVANCES made during the early part of the 20th century, reconstructive surgeons couldn't keep pace with the large numbers of wounded soldiers. M. Alphonse Louis was not the only one to emerge from combat as a masked man. Some wartime injuries were simply too extensive to be repaired, so hiding them became the next-best option.

In England, a sculptor named Francis Derwent Wood found himself a unique niche. He began his military service as an orderly but was overcome by the number of soldiers with ghastly facial wounds. Many of these soldiers committed suicide; others were afraid to return home, and one could only guess their fates. These men faced the enemy and the savagery of war with grit, yet they were too ashamed of their appearance to face the people who loved them.

Wood opened a workshop in a London hospital to create masks for disfigured soldiers. Inside the Masks for Facial Disfigurements Department (informally, the department was called the Tin Noses Shop), Wood created masks of silver-plated electroplate. Using oil paints, he painted the masks to look like the soldiers, using prewar photographs. He added glass eyes and facial hair made of thin strands of silver. Hidden behind a mask, a disfigured soldier could at least feel confident enough to walk down the street, meet a stranger, and return home to his family. At Sidcup a few masks were made, but their owners hated them, and as reconstruction became more competent, masks were largely abandoned.

Before the War to End All Wars, there was little need for masks of metal. But throughout history, people have lost eyes or noses to disease or injury. Physicians have always been forced to be innovative to help those with missing parts look as whole as possible.

※

CHAPTER 5

the dog ate my eye

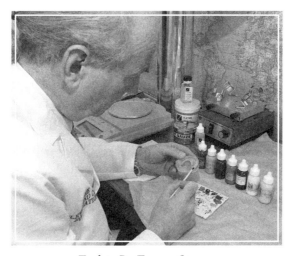

The late Dr. Thomas Cowper

The face is often only a smooth imposter.

—Pierre Corneille

"I AVOID COCKTAIL PARTIES. People just don't understand," said Dr. Thomas Cowper. When he wasn't dodging social invitations, Dr. Cowper, who died unexpectedly in 2007, was typically holed up in a small lab at Cleveland Clinic, creating ears, noses, and combinations of facial parts for people who had lost their originals. Although it might sound as though he didn't like talking about his work, he did. He considered it a serious endeavor.

It is believed that thousands of years ago, Egyptians replaced lost ears with duplicates fashioned from wax. If you lost your nose in China, it may have been replaced with another made from wax or wood. Between the second and 16th centuries, facial prostheses, mainly ears and noses, were fashioned from all sorts of material — from enameled gold, silver, and porcelain to leather, wax, resin, wood, clay, and, if you were very poor, papier-mâché. (One can only imagine how poorly a nose of papier-mâché would perform on a rainy day.)

Paintings from the 16th century show the Danish astronomer Tycho Brahe wearing a prosthetic nose made from metal. According to history, a swift slice of an enemy sword stole part of his nose. (The ability to lop off your opponent's nose was a sign of superb swordsmanship.) It is believed that Brahe sported a nasal prosthesis made from gold and silver for special occasions and another of a heavier metal for everyday use.

Today, facial prostheses are made from medical-grade silicone, which offers the wearer comfort and a reasonably natural look. Most facial prostheses are created by anaplastologists, specialists trained in making facial and body prostheses, and maxillofacial (maxilla means "jaw") prosthodontists, dentists specially trained in developing prostheses for the head and neck. Prosthetic eyes are the product of specialists called ocularists.

Dr. Cowper, who routinely wore his thinning silver-streaked hair in a ponytail, was a trained maxillofacial prosthodontist; he headed Cleveland Clinic's Section of Maxillofacial Prosthetics, a unique dental subspecialty. Roughly 260 physicians belong to the American Academy of Maxillofacial Prosthetics; 100 or fewer practice clinically in the United States.

Many physicians and medical centers shy away from the subspecialty because of low insurance reimbursement. Facial prostheses are expensive to create; a nose, for example, can cost up to $7,000, for which Medicare and Medicaid might reimburse the physician only $1,500.

Dr. Salvatore Esposito, who chaired Cleveland Clinic's Department of Dentistry for years and now is in private practice, says the need for facial prostheses is decreasing for two reasons. One is that because of combined therapy for cancer — surgery, radiation, and chemotherapy — less initial damage is done to patients; thus, many are able to escape disfiguring surgery. "In the past, a surgeon would simply remove the tumor. What was left was up to someone else to fix," he says.

The second reason is that because of advances in plastic and reconstructive surgery, injuries that would have required a facial prosthesis are now repaired in the operating room. "Surgeons are so adept at putting patients back together again," says Dr. Esposito.

Nevertheless, some patients are a poor surgical risk or are unwilling to undergo reconstructive surgery — most often multiple surgeries, depending on the extent of their injury — so they opt for a prosthesis.

WHEN MATTHEW MCGRATH'S grandson, also named Matthew, was about eight years old, he was convinced that "Grampy" was a pirate. The older Matthew wears a piece of Velcro the size of an eye patch over the area of his right eye. Another piece of Velcro fits onto the first piece and wraps around his head. Together, they work to hold a plastic insert that fits over the right side of Matthew's face. "A friend of mine calls it a mask, and, in a sense, that's true. It matches the other side of my face," he explains.

In 1983, Matthew was told he had sinus cancer. The disease started in his right maxillary, or cheekbone. His team of head and neck surgeons performed a dozen or so surgeries on him and then referred him to Cleveland Clinic because "I had a large hole in my head," says Matthew, who was fifty at the time.

He describes the damage to his face like this: Put your thumb on your right ear and your pinkie finger on your nose. Then extend your fingers to the upper portion of your eyebrow and press the bottom of your hand on your jawbone. That section of his face is missing. "It's quite large," he says. So large, in fact, that it took several long appointments to create the prosthesis and then hours and hours of detail work to make it look just right.

Early on, Matthew asked Dr. Esposito why it took him so long to finesse the prosthesis; after all, he'd heard about a woman who'd had a knee replacement and had walked out of the hospital within a matter of days.

"He looked at me and wasn't quite sure if he should answer me honestly or not," Matthew says, "and I could see he almost shrugged his shoulders, as if to say, 'Aw, hell.' So his answer was 'The other guys get more practice than I do.' Then he explained that people who had my problem were usually dead before he got to see them!"

Matthew's prosthesis was fashioned from acrylic and, because it's so large, made hollow to keep it as lightweight as possible. Dr. Esposito admits that he tried to "get fancy" with Matthew's prosthesis at first, wanting to include an artificial eye and a beard to match the other side of his face, but Matthew wanted to keep it simple. Function was his priority: He simply wanted to be able to speak and eat.

Matthew is missing his upper and lower jaw on his right side, as well as all his teeth. To give him the most function, Dr. Esposito fitted him with a denture that replaces the missing portion of his lower right jaw and fits over the remaining part of his lower left jaw. He then created an upper denture for the right side that is attached to Matthew's facial prosthesis. With his prosthesis on, Matthew can speak in a way that is understandable and he is able to eat. With the prosthesis off, however, he loses both those abilities.

If Matthew were to have similar cancer surgery today, his outcome might be different. Dr. Esposito explains that years ago, when people lost part of their lower jaw, they were often left with a devastating deformity. The jaw would shift to one side, giving the lower face a crooked appearance. Surgeons now use microvascular free flaps to reconstruct the jaw right at the time of cancer surgery. Usually, the surgeons use a bone from the leg (fibula), the peroneal artery, and smaller veins, along with any tissue if needed. The bone is shaped to fit the defect and attached to a reconstruction plate. The bone and plate are then inserted into the jaw, and the artery and blood vessels are attached to the existing blood supply.

Repairing an upper jaw, however, is a horse of a different color, says Dr. Esposito. Upper-jaw repairs can be successful from a medical standpoint, but they are a nightmare from a functional one. A better solution for the patient is to be fitted with an obturator, a prosthesis that fits inside the mouth to allow eating and speaking.

Matthew doesn't seem bothered much about his disfigurement. He says the people who have problems with him usually are adults. "It's hard for them to look at me without feeling some sense of sorrow. Or, sometimes, surprise."

A couple of years ago, Matthew and his wife, Janet, were on a cruise. For dinner, they were seated with two African-American couples and a white couple. Later, the white couple admitted to the McGraths that when they first saw the African-American couples approaching the table, they thought they might feel uncomfortable. "Then they saw me coming!" Matthew says with a laugh.

Unlike adults, children seem to be more accepting of differences. "They don't have any problem with me," says Matthew. "Young children accept me for what I am."

Some years ago, Matthew and Janet were grocery shopping, and a young girl riding in the grocery cart looked up at Matthew and asked, "Hey, mister, what happened to your face?"

Matthew responded, "I had a boo-boo."

"I have a boo-boo, too!" the girl shared. Then off came her shoe and she showed Matthew the blister on her heel.

Rather than social interactions, the most challenging adjustment for Matthew was his inability to work. He had taught statistics and computer technology at a university and then worked for the government. Eventually, he started his own business, which involved training programs.

"I was a teacher, spent most of my life teaching, and spoke clearly and never had any problem being understood. At least until this cancer. I couldn't work because I couldn't talk. It was a big adjustment." Matthew, now in his seventies, says, "I still think or dream about teaching classes."

Despite all the surgeries and having to live differently because of his prosthesis, Matthew is simply grateful for survival. His ordeal wasn't easy, but he was willing to go through it because he didn't want to die. "I was supposed to have been dead within six to eight months," recalls Matthew, "and that was more than twenty years ago."

Today, Matthew sees Dr. Esposito once or twice a year to get his prosthesis fine-tuned. Sometimes, Dr. Esposito will find a better way of attaching the device so it doesn't slip off as easily. Every now and again, he'll create a new one, because they don't last forever.

Matthew is grateful that Dr. Esposito was able to help him. He jokes, "If I saw somebody with a hole in his head the size of mine, and this person was asking me to do something about it, I'd run for the nearest door!"

FACIAL PROSTHESES ARE tailor-made for each patient. "Each is distinct; all are challenging from not only a functional perspective, but also a cosmetic one. It's difficult getting something artificial to look natural. Getting the right shape and color is challenging," said Dr. Cowper.

The color of human skin is affected by the way light hits it. Real skin is made up of layers of varying types of pigment that contain beta-carotene, melanin, and hemoglobin. Matching skin color is not as easy as picking a paint chip and asking the guy behind the counter to mix up a quart.

Naturally, a missing ear is made to match the remaining ear (including holes for earrings), but with noses, there's more flexibility. For example, when Dr. Cowper created a prosthetic nose, he talked to his patients about how they wanted their new nose to look. He also relied on photographs of people before their injuries.

Asked if women were pickier about a new nose than men, Dr. Cowper said, "Both men and women are picky about their new nose. It's probably the only time they have a chance to have exactly what they want." Creating a nose is most challenging because it's the first thing one sees on the face. The nose also is typically the first facial feature to be damaged, particularly by skin cancer. Its prominence on the face is likely to blame, attracting all sorts of attention — good and bad. The nose is a lightning rod, a mad golfer swinging away in a thunderstorm.

A facial prosthesis will generally last about five years; if the piece gets a lot of sun exposure, it has a shorter life. It's not uncommon for people to have prostheses for different seasons. A summer ear will be a darker shade than a winter ear, for example.

Because reconstructive surgery on ears is not extremely successful, prosthetic ears are common. "Ears are complicated structures to totally re-create," said Dr. Cowper. "By and large, most surgeons aren't able to correct an ear to look the way a prosthetic ear can look." An attempt at growing an ear on the back of a mouse was only somewhat successful; researchers involved in tissue engineering are working furiously to remedy that.

Prosthetic ears are typically affixed using an implant system called bony implants, similar to the type used for dental implants. Small screws are implanted into the skull where the ear should be. Once the bone heals around the screws, a structure made from metal and gold is attached to the screws. The prosthetic ear then clips onto the structure.

A prosthesis affixed with implant technology generally gives the wearer extra reassurance. With implants, the chances of the prosthesis slipping or falling off are slim.

Care of a facial prosthesis is straightforward. The piece is washed with soap and water and taken off at night to give the facial tissues a chance to rest. Besides, the sticking power of adhesives, used to affix most prostheses to the face, doesn't last that long. After a whole day, the glue is ready to let go.

People with facial prostheses don't have any real restrictions. Swimming or participating in sports isn't out of the question. "Each person has his or her own tolerances, so they learn what they are. You start out slowly and adjust. It's an ongoing process," said Dr. Cowper.

About a third of Dr. Cowper's workday was spent in the lab, creating facial prostheses. The lab is tiny and warm, courtesy of the lineup of Bunsen burners shooting eight-inch flames. (Superficial burns on the forearms are common.) At any given time, five or six professionals are seated around a wooden worktable that takes up much of the room. Shelves of colorful plastic bins hold an assortment of ears and noses.

Creating a prosthesis is a complex, painstaking endeavor, requiring patience and multiple office visits on the part of the patient and skill and long hours in the laboratory on the part of the professional. First, an impression of the area to be fitted is made. If the prosthesis is an ear, an impression of the remaining ear is taken. Next, a cast is made from the impression, from which a wax model is then created. If the model is acceptable to the patient, an acrylic version is made.

A nose takes about 12 hours to create. A larger piece — say, half a face and an ear — could take between 20 and 30 hours. Once a piece is created, it is taken to the prosthodontist's office, which often resembles an art studio. Tabletops are littered with dozens of paint bottles containing vibrant colors and variations of flesh tones. Paper palettes and bouquets of paintbrushes in jars compete for space.

If a swath of hair is needed, such as an eyebrow, one is fashioned using synthetic hair placed on a backing and affixed to the prosthesis.

A sample eyebrow looks somewhat like an anchovy. If just a few hairs are needed — around the ear canal, for example — single synthetic hairs are plugged into the prosthesis using a pick-like instrument and a shot of glue.

To the professional, the prostheses never look real enough. The color isn't quite right or the finished shape is too bumpy. But, more often than not, the people who need these parts welcome them with open arms. When patients apply their prostheses and look at themselves in the mirror, they don't seem to notice an uneven edge or a minor variation in color. They just see themselves as whole again.

The most successful patients are accepting in nature. "They have reasonable self-esteem and accept their injury, yet they realize still nothing has changed internally," said Dr. Cowper. "Most people are like that. Humans are extremely resilient. As we go through life, most people accept situations better than you'd think. There are a few people who are angry and resentful, but I haven't seen many."

A TECHNIQUE BORROWED FROM industrial design, with applications in the auto and toy industries, is being used to help create facial prostheses and to assist surgeons when they're planning reconstructive surgeries. Called rapid prototyping, the technique involves taking ultrathin slices of two-dimensional computerized tomography (CT) scans or magnetic resonance (MR) scans of a skull, for example, and creating a solid three-dimensional version, an actual plastic model.

Using sophisticated software, Angela Noecker, a senior research engineer at the Cleveland Clinic Lerner Research Institute, highlights the portions of the scanned images from which she wants to create a model. She selects certain pixels, based on gray values, with an eye toward capturing specific bony structures that will be included in a three-dimensional on-screen model.

When the on-screen model looks accurate to her and the consulting surgeon, she outputs the information to the rapid prototyping device, also called a stereolithography machine. The lower part of the device is a vat filled with liquid photopolymer, a viscous material a little thinner than honey. Covering the vat of liquid is a screen, upon which the three-dimensional model will rest once it is created. The upper part of the device is a laser, directed at the liquid.

Once the information is downloaded, the device begins to draw the model, using ultraviolet laser and photochemistry technology. The laser traces a cross section of the model layer by layer. After a layer is drawn, the liquid photopolymer hardens, and the screen drops just about a third of a millimeter into the liquid. Another layer is drawn, and the screen drops again. After several hours, depending on the size of the piece, the result is an anatomically accurate three-dimensional model. "It takes about eighteen to twenty-four hours for a skull," says Noecker. "A jaw takes between five and six hours."

Although the technology is typically used for creating models of bony structures, such as a jaw, Noecker and her colleagues experimented with creating models of soft tissue — skin and muscle — thinking it might help reconstructive surgeons with more difficult cases. If the surgeon wants a flexible version of a soft-tissue model, one can be created in the polymer laboratory. Molds are made from the plastic models and, from those, flexible models made from silicone or polyurethane are created.

Let's say a woman is having facial reconstruction on the right side of her face because of an accident. The eye socket and cheekbone on her right side have been badly damaged, and she's lost a lot of tissue from that area. The left side of her face is unscathed. A mold is made of her entire face. From that mold, Noecker can create a rigid model of the woman's skull, which will show how much work needs to be done to repair her damaged eye socket and cheekbone. She also can create a mirror image of the woman's good side, from which a mold can be made. Using the mold, a flexible model can be created, which the surgeon can use to determine how much soft tissue is required to build up the right side of her face.

Using the models during facial reconstruction surgery helps eliminate guesswork. Rather than having to rely on an estimate for how much bone and soft tissue a patient might need, based on traditional two-dimensional imaging scans, the models offer an exact plan in a user-friendly format.

Physicians also use the models to help with diagnosis, to measure bone displacement, and to shape implants. Using this type of model allows them to determine the thickness of a bone, so they have a better idea of where to place a prosthesis, such as an ear or nose. The only facial prosthetic Cleveland Clinic doesn't make is eyes. Said Dr. Cowper, "There simply are too many good ocularists out there."

DARRELL HARDIN GREETS PEOPLE with his boyish smile and hands them a chocolate and caramel eye, genuine eye candy. Although this good-natured prank is usually reserved for his youngest patients, he says that some of his male adult patients also enjoy the candy. His female patients? As much as they may love chocolate, many don't appreciate the prank quite the same way. It's the eye part, you understand. Too personal. Too relevant.

Hardin is a certified ocular anaplastologist. He makes and fits artificial eyes for people who were born without them, or who lost them to injury or illness. But he's not your typical medical professional. His eyes and his grin are the first clues. He's often more like a little kid in a grownup's body, with a grownup's job. For instance, he has a lot of fun with patients' typical reaction to his putting in their artificial eyes for the first time.

"They open their mouths!" he laughs. "'Am I feeding a bird?' I say. 'Why are you opening your mouth? I'm not putting the eye in there!'"

And he, of course, knows all the eye jokes: A guy who swallowed his eye goes to the proctologist and crawls up onto the table. The doctor takes a look with the scope and says, "My God, in twenty-five years of looking at these things, this is the first time I've had one look back!" He admits the jokes are bad, but the jokes, the silly banter, and the playfulness are really tools to help patients relax.

Underneath Hardin's wackiness is a genuine, compassionate man. He joined the U.S. Navy as a young man and served as a corpsman with the Field Medical Force during Vietnam. In conjunction with the University of Missouri, St. Louis, he trained with the U.S. Department of Medicine and Surgery and the Veterans Administration. He worked with the head-and-neck oral surgery team as an operating-room scrub, taking care of the injured soldiers who were flown home. "In the seventies, there was quite a pool of people with injuries," he says.

His very first case involved a young man (Hardin still remembers his full name) who took a point-blank shot to the lower left side of his face. The exit wound was on the right side of his face. Hardin's boss, a Navy captain, instructed him to unwrap the patient's bandages, debride (clean) the wound, and evaluate the injuries. "Might as well get your feet wet," he said to Hardin.

"His head was half-wrapped in a large piece of gauze. His uncovered eye was open and looking around. I explained to him what I was going to do. I unwrapped the gauze and gasped," he says. Half the young man's face had been destroyed, and he was missing his right eye. Part of the man's brain, the frontal lobe, was exposed. "My knees were shaking, my hands were quivering, and I was nauseated," says Hardin. That young man survived, but many others didn't.

Hardin has been making eyes for 30 years, and he says he can't even begin to guess how many eyes that might be. He has the first eye he ever made, even though his boss at the time insisted he throw it away, and he has three boxes of "bad" eyes, eyes that didn't quite pass muster.

"My mood reflects in the eye," he says. If he's feeling sharp, the eye will reflect it. Sometimes an eye will look cloudy to him. "The crispness isn't there," he says. Those eyes go in one of the boxes.

Each patient gets at least two artificial eyes, one and an extra. He explains that most patients need to have an extra eye handy because they disappear. "They really do," he nods, explaining that the eye socket is not much more than a mucous membrane. Plastic, being porous, absorbs the enzymes in the body, giving the eyes an organic odor attractive to animals, particularly those of the canine variety. "Dogs eat them," he says. "Cats, they just bat them around."

Hundreds of years ago, ocular prostheses were fashioned from leather, silk, metal, and animal hides. As early as the fifth century B.C., artificial eyes were made from clay and fastened to the outside of the eye socket with cloth. In the 16th century, the Venetians used glass to make ocular prostheses that fit inside the eye. A German craftsman named Ludwig Muller-Uri was the first to make prosthetic eyes from cryolite glass, the same material he used to make doll eyes. The practice of making ocular prostheses from glass continued until after World War II, when the U.S. Army's Dental Department created the first plastic eyes.

Today's ocular prostheses are made from acrylic, and the method is nearly the same as creating a facial prosthesis. First, an impression of the eye socket is made to determine the size and shape of the artificial eye. From the impression, a wax model is created. Using the model, an ocularist decides where the iris should be painted and how the prosthesis will fit into the eye. The wax model is then painted under a special light that simulates north-sky daylight, and it is packed into acrylic and heated at a high temperature to cure the acrylic. Tinfoil in the molds draws out the uncured poison naturally found in acrylic. Hardin uses an adapted version of a curing technique, developed for dentures by a Mexican dentist. He microwaves the eyes.

Finally, the finishing touches are put on the eye. Hardin still has a 1920s spool of Chinese red silk thread that he was given 30 years ago. He shreds the very end of the thread to get tiny, fine silk fibers that are used to mimic naturally occurring veins in the eye. The similarity is amazing, perhaps even more so because over the years the thread has faded unevenly, giving the fibers an even more realistic look. The eye is then smoothed with a grinder to remove scratches or irritants.

Contrary to what one might imagine, artificial eyes are not full orbits like a natural eye. They are more like shells that fit over the natural eye or that fit over an implant placed in the socket where an orbit used to be. They look like long fake nails.

Hardin's patient base is wide, and he typically has between 50 and 60 new patients at any given time. He's caring for a total of about 4,000 right now. Most of his patients are sent from the U.S. State Department. He also creates prosthetic eyes for prisoners, veterans, international dignitaries, and people from across the country and from around the world who learn of his skill via the Internet. Ocularists are in high demand. Hardin says there are about 306 of them in all, and the American Society of Ocularists reports about 220 members.

A true artist, Hardin sculpts and paints in his spare time. Although being an ocularist can be challenging, frustrating, and sometimes downright depressing — he's had some heartbreaking cases — he admits that he's good at what he does. "Patients are willing to do anything to look 'normal,' to a degree. So, if you have a God-given talent, how can you not use it?" he asks.

He closely identifies with his patients, possibly because he's been in the business a long time but more likely because three of his family members — mother, brother, and stepdaughter — have artificial eyes. (What are the odds?)

He takes great care to get to know his patients before even beginning to try to help them. "Each person is a complication with a situation," he says. "We'll spend an hour just talking." Ordinarily, even with children, that part of his job is easy. Working more and more with an international clientele, however, has added some cultural and communication challenges.

"I had an Islamic woman as a patient, and I couldn't look in her eyes," he explains, referring to the custom that prohibits a strange man from making eye contact with a married woman. "I was not allowed to talk to her and not allowed to stare into her eyes," he says. Hardin had to try to communicate through the woman's husband, brother-in-law, and parents.

While he was fitting her new eye, she suddenly raised her arm to her eye as if it hurt. Hardin asked whether she was having pain. "She's okay," her husband said, without bothering to ask his wife. This went on for a while until Hardin was able to convince them that if she had pain, it would only get worse. Finally, the husband asked his wife if she had pain, and she told him where it hurt.

"The women are not allowed to express pain; they're told to shut up," says Hardin. "But I needed to know whether there was discomfort because it could lead to infection. That was a rough one to do."

Through the years, he's had some unusual requests. His VA patients have asked him to paint a variety of images on their eyes, usually right where the pupil would be. They've asked for Playboy bunnies, breasts, and the Harley-Davidson logo. Women tend to be more reserved, but he has been asked a few times to put a diamond in the pupil.

"Bring me the diamond, I'll put it in!" he laughs, happy to add a little sparkle to someone's eye.

For children, he often paints an image on the top part of the prosthesis that helps them identify which way it goes in. The image is hidden by their eyelid. Butterflies are a favorite among his young female patients.

He once was asked to help one of his patients after the patient had died. The man had lost a large part of his face and eye to cancer, but the family wanted an open casket for the wake. So Hardin went to the funeral home and worked on the gentleman's eye.

"I sat down there with a heat gun until two in the morning," says Hardin, when he got to the point where he could put the eyelashes on. Then he helped the undertaker put the man in his coffin and close it.

Hardin lights a cigarette and offers a prosthetic eye that had been made by someone else for a person who didn't have insurance or enough money to self-pay. "Can you see the difference?" he asks, comparing it to a prosthetic eye that he created. The first eye is murky, oddly colored, and without depth. It looks as though it might even belong to a second-rate doll. The eye made from Hardin's handiwork is nothing short of extraordinary. The eye centered in the palm appears living and the hand becomes an ancient amulet, a powerful fetish, capable of warding off evil.

The difference is remarkable enough to make Hardin angry. These people deserve better, he says, especially when you realize their circumstances. Describing the mindset of many of his patients, he says, "I was born this way. I didn't ask for it. I didn't volunteer.'"

He's right. All of them were called on a journey and had to make the trip, whether they wanted to or not.

CHAPTER 6

little prizefighter

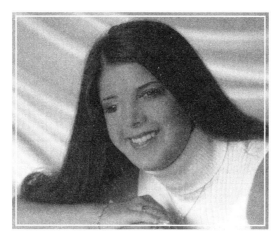

Melissa Wallace

*You gain strength, courage, and confidence
by each experience in which you really
stop to look fear in the face.*

—Eleanor Roosevelt

AUTUMN IN NORTHEAST OHIO, as in other northern climes, is a time when nature begins to ready itself for winter. The earth prepares to accept what will not survive by softening, so it can consume the tall sunflowers of summer and dry leaves of fall that rain down from the sky like confetti. All that dies goes back to the earth, enveloped in soil and composted. The smell is ancient, pungent. As winter nears, the landscape quiets. The animals of the year — kits, poults, fawns, and cubs — hunker down in preparation for frigid temperatures and lack of food. Only the strongest live.

In the fall of 1984, Debbie Hardin was preparing for the birth of her third child. The trees were just starting to turn. On the morning she went into labor, her then husband, Tom, was attending early mass. When he returned home, he drove Debbie the 30 miles to Mt. Sinai Hospital in Cleveland, leaving their other two children, Tom Jr. and Kim, in a neighbor's care.

At the hospital, Debbie's obstetrician was helping to pass the time by telling Debbie about a new doctor they'd just hired. He was a plastic surgeon, very well known, and the hospital was lucky to recruit him, he said. His name was Dr. Bahman Guyuron.

At 9:36 A.M., on September 16, Debbie gave birth to a seven-pound, eight-ounce baby girl. They named her Melissa. She had a full head of dark hair, just as her older brother and sister did when they were born. But before Debbie could even see or hold her new daughter, the baby was whisked away by the nurses.

She recalls her doctor telling her, "It's okay. I'm friends with this guy," referring to Dr. Guyuron. "I'll have him here in the morning."

After she delivered, Debbie was moved to a private room and left to wonder about the fate of her baby. "I had a little girl with facial defects. That's all I knew," says Debbie. "I was wondering if she was okay, how bad it was."

Hours would pass before she was able to hold Melissa. Even then, Debbie would have her only long enough to see that her right eyelid wouldn't open, her nose and right ear were deformed, and her skull appeared to be formed incorrectly.

MELISSA WAS BORN WITH hemifacial microsomia, the most common facial birth defect after clefts. Hemifacial refers to half of the face and microsomia means small structures. Thus, children born with hemifacial microsomia typically have underdeveloped features on one half of their face. Most often the jaw, mouth, and ear (sometimes internally as well as externally, which results in hearing loss) are affected. Sometimes the skull, eye and eye socket, and cheek are affected. The affected half of the face is shorter than the unaffected side, making the face asymmetrical, or uneven. When the skull is involved, as it was in Melissa's case, intracranial surgery sometimes is necessary to ensure the brain has enough room to grow normally.

Melissa also was born with Tessier clefts 2 and 7. A cleft is a gap in tissue or bone; some are much more severe than others. Tessier clefts (named after French plastic surgeon Dr. Paul Tessier) are more complex than the more common cleft lip and cleft palate, involving other areas of the face. They are numbered 0 to 14 to describe their location on the face. A Tessier cleft 2 involves the outer curve of the nostril and the top of the lip. A Tessier cleft 7 gives the mouth a wide appearance and involves the cheekbone, the side of the face, the ear, and the lower eyelid. Repair of Tessier clefts is surgically challenging, because often the clefts involve both soft tissue and bone.

One half of Melissa's face was unaffected; the other side appeared to be somewhat shrunken, with a ridge cutting across all the affected areas. Her right eye was the size of a shriveled pea and, naturally, would never function. Her right ear was deformed; the lobe developed low and clung to her jaw. The nerves on the right side of her face were not in the usual areas.

The good news was that the results from X-rays and CT scans taken right after she was born were normal; the rest of her anatomy appeared to be okay. Melissa did not have brain damage. Other than her craniofacial conditions, she was a perfectly healthy, strong baby.

Like Debbie's two previous pregnancies, this one had been uneventful. She took excellent care of herself, avoiding all medications, alcohol, and caffeine. She took her vitamins and folic acid like clockwork. The usual rounds of ultrasounds showed no abnormalities or reasons for concern. There was no reason to suspect that her baby would be born in any condition less than "perfect."

Still, like any parent in that situation, Debbie was focused on what she might have done wrong to cause this. She asked herself, "What did I do? What did I eat? I wondered if it was because of microwave cooking—this was about the time microwaves came out. It sounds silly, but I was looking for answers," she says. Nothing made sense.

"Everyone was just in shock because it was so unexpected," says Debbie, remembering how alone she felt after Melissa was born. Her parents came to the hospital to see her and the baby. Her father said to her, "It's going to be a long road."

Debbie remembers Tom's reaction to seeing Melissa for the first time. "He said, 'You call everyone and tell them what you had.' And then he left."

DR. ROBERT NASEEF IS a private-practice psychologist in Philadelphia. He specializes in working with families with special-needs children and has expertise in the psychology of men, particularly fathers.

When a baby is born with a disability, most often the father does not reject the child, says Dr. Naseef, but a handful of fathers, for whatever reason, cannot cope. They may feel angry, guilty, ashamed, or some combination of emotions that cause them to turn away and retreat.

"Generally, among parents of kids with disabilities, there's a continuum. Some are overprotective and that's the one extreme; the other extreme is rejection. It's the extreme, but it is in the range of what happens," he says. "People with disabilities experience rejection. Hopefully, it's not with a parent, but rejection is part of the experience and kids will need to learn to cope with it as part of their developmental process. This takes time and a child certainly needs support to deal with this extremely painful emotion."

Unlike women, men generally find it difficult to talk about something they can't fix or control. When a child is born with a disability, it can be enough to throw a father into a complete tailspin. "If we can't fix it, we tend not to want to talk about it. Most fathers of kids with a disability have a similar feeling, but many fathers overcome some or all of that," explains Dr. Naseef, who himself has a child with autism.

This is why support for the family is crucial from the moment a baby with disabilities is born. Hospitals should make every effort to connect new parents with other parents of children with disabilities for support, he says. "And there's a special value in a man talking with another man."

Typically, though, many medical professionals are more comfortable talking to the mother. Dr. Naseef gives the example of a pediatrician who calls the house. When the father answers the phone, the doctor asks to speak to the mother. Men are sort of factored out from the beginning, he says, so when tragedy happens, why do we think they'll factor in?

"The assumption is the woman will deal with it — will deal with the school, will deal with the doctor," he says. Part of the reason is that women possess a stronger instinct to nurture, whereas men are programmed or expected to be providers and protectors. When a situation is complicated, the same man who was factored out when the situation was ordinary is suddenly thrust into the fray. The man can't fix the problem, so he doesn't know how to talk about it. He feels unable to help and unless he can find the language to talk about how he's feeling, he may feel unable to cope. In that case, his reaction may be to withdraw emotionally, physically, or both.

Positive adjustments within families can happen, says Dr. Naseef, particularly if the medical community makes the effort to talk to parents together about their children. "As the father gets comfortable talking about the disability, it helps the whole family," he says. "If Dad talks about it, then it's okay to talk about it."

Even with the absence of her father, Melissa's support system was strong and stable. From the time she was born until today, 22 years later, she's been surrounded by her mother, sister, and brother. Dr. Guyuron and his nurse, Theresa Thomas, also have been caring for Melissa since she was born.

"She had a very, very supportive mother who stood by her side all the time. Unfortunately, that doesn't happen all the time. There are families that fall apart; there are parents who abandon children. Debbie was there all the time. She did a superb job," says Dr. Guyuron.

Being there and knowing what to do didn't always come easy. "It was a long road," says Debbie, referring to her father's words to her when Melissa was born. "He was right."

ONE YEAR RIGHT BEFORE Christmas, Debbie and Melissa were shopping to pick up a few last-minute gifts. Melissa, then just two years old, was enchanted with the colors and lights of the season. The twinkling lights that challenge December's long nights and the smell of fresh pine boughs are reminders that the darkest, coldest season is halfway over. The holiday proposes the notion that everyone should be just a little kinder, a little more generous, and a little more thoughtful.

Holding a gift in one hand and steering Melissa's stroller with the other, Debbie made her way into the checkout line. In line in front of them were two women who had noticed Melissa right away. After staring at her for a few seconds, both women turned around. With her other two children, Debbie would have heard how darling her baby was or how cute she looked; everyone loves to fuss over small children. They would have asked her name or how old she was, and Debbie would have beamed. Instead, with their backs to Debbie, one woman said to the other, "That's just awful. Her mother must have been on drugs or alcohol."

With tears welling in her eyes, Debbie dropped the gift, turned

Melissa's stroller around, and hurried out of the store. Safe in her car, she sat and cried. "I didn't know how to cope," she says.

MELISSA UNDERWENT HER first surgery when she was five months old and her last when she was 19 years old. Over the course of years, Dr. Guyuron rebuilt her forehead, where she was missing some bone, by repositioning her own bone and using layers of bone grafts taken from her hip. He expanded her eye socket with an implant, using better materials as they became available. He repositioned her eyebrow and closed the cleft in her nose. He then lengthened Melissa's upper and lower jaws.

Some surgeries were to smooth out prior procedures or to correct abnormal growth in the skull and face. A procedure may offer a satisfactory result until the child grows again, the growth resulting in imperfections or flaws that require correction, says Dr. Guyuron, who today is the chief of Plastic and Reconstructive Surgery at University Hospitals Case Medical Center.

All told, Melissa has had 42 surgeries, including three cranial surgeries, in 19 years. Her mother has been at her side each time.

"I was always there, and I cried every time. All forty-two times. It's hard to put your child to sleep," says Debbie. Every time Melissa was wheeled into the operating room, Debbie would walk away clutching Lambie, Melissa's favorite stuffed animal. Lambie was given to Melissa before her first surgery; it went through all the surgeries with her, usually wearing a hospital wristband before surgery and an eye patch afterward.

Melissa's childhood was wrapped tightly in bandages and held in the hands of doctors and nurses. The days, months, and years collected in the corners of the operating rooms and beneath recovery-room beds until they were swept up and tossed away. The smell of disinfectant embedded itself in the recesses of her mind, so that years later simply walking through the front entrance of a medical center would cause her to faint.

MOST OF THE SURGERIES Melissa has undergone have been to rebuild her right eye socket, so that she could be fitted with a prosthetic eye. Bone was taken from her groin area and grafted to the socket, without full success because of partial absorption of the graft. Dr. Guyuron tried using coralline hydroxyapatite, which is a material derived from coral, to build up her eye socket. Unlike other materials, it is resistant to infection and has a high biocompatibility, which means the body is unlikely to reject it. Frustrated with the results of Melissa's eye surgeries, Dr. Guyuron wishes there were a better way. The intent is there; the science is not.

When Melissa was five, Debbie took her to see Darrell Hardin, an ocularist in Cleveland, to inquire about a prosthetic eye. Hardin remembers that Melissa's eye socket was filled with soft tissue, so there wasn't enough room for an artificial eye. Furthermore, her socket was susceptible to bouts of infections. By the time Melissa saw Hardin, she had already lost her right eyelid and lashes to infection. There are three requirements for bacteria to grow: moisture, darkness, and warmth, explains Hardin. A tiny, empty eye socket meets all those requirements. "If you break up the trilogy, then bacteria can't grow," he says.

Hardin fitted Melissa with a clear pressure conformer, which is an oval-shaped piece of acrylic that fits into the eye socket. He made Melissa's conformer clear to let in light and dry the moisture, so that the inside of her eye could heal and the cycles of infection could stop. The conformer also works to stretch and push back scar tissue in preparation for an artificial eye.

"Tissue and bone are pliable," says Hardin. "If you give continuous pressure to tissue, not to the point of necrosis, but increase pressure slowly and regularly, you can move tissue around." If nothing is placed inside an empty eye socket, the tissue and bone eventually will grow over the opening. But if something appropriate is placed inside, it stimulates growth, acting "almost like an irritant," he says, and is safe as long as it doesn't cause infection.

Hardin's recommendation for wearing the conformer was specific.

Despite what conventional wisdom said, he was sure that this particular combination of pressure and time would allow the socket to open and heal. If it did, Melissa would avoid more surgeries to accomplish the same goal. Debbie followed the instructions religiously, he says, keeping a log of everything, including any issues she identified. She noticed right away whether the tissue below the eye was turning white, which meant it wasn't getting blood because of the pressure. "The lines of communication were kept wide open," he says. "If there was a problem, they came right in." Slowly, Melissa's socket began to open, and the infections cleared once and for all.

The day before Thanksgiving that year, Debbie asked Hardin to make a tiny eye for Melissa so that she would have it for the holiday. At the time, Hardin says Melissa's socket was still in bad shape. The tissue was thick, and they'd just gotten to the point where they could insert a tiny conformer. Debbie asked him whether he could just add some color to the conformer — paint a little iris to make it look like an eye. So he crafted a small brown eye, the size of a little-finger fingernail, and fitted it for Melissa. He stepped back to take a look.

Shaking his head, he said, "No, no, no, this is not what we're looking for." But Debbie wouldn't hear it. She stood back, looked at Melissa, and cried. "You don't understand," she told Hardin. "This is the first time in my baby's life that she's looking back at me."

He understood. "She hurt so bad," he says.

On Thanksgiving Day, Debbie made sure all her guests saw Melissa's new eye. "It didn't look pretty to a soul but to me," says Debbie. "I looked at my daughter and she was looking back at me with two eyes. That was all I wanted." Her daughter was whole.

About the time Melissa finished the first grade, her father left. Four years later, her mother and father's divorce was final. The following year, when Melissa was about 11, Debbie and Darrell Hardin married. Although their marriage later ended, they are still constants in each other's lives and Hardin still refers to Melissa as "my girl." When Melissa was small, he would hold her close — she burying the right side of her face, her "bad" side, into his leg — and for a few minutes, at least, he was able to give her solace and remind her that she was loved very much. Healer, guardian, and protector, this father didn't — and won't ever — budge.

MOST IMPROVEMENTS TO Melissa's face were directly related to functional issues. They were performed to keep her brain from being crushed by her skull, to help her breathe, and to allow her to chew properly. Many of the surgeries, however, also improved her appearance, realigning her features and giving her face symmetry.

Debbie always thought each surgery was an improvement. She would meet Melissa in the recovery room after surgery and gaze down at her, able to see the results through the rows of black stitches and dried blood. Days later, Debbie says, the swelling would take over, causing Melissa to look like a "little prizefighter." But before the swelling crept through Melissa's tissues, enveloping her face, Debbie would stand at her bedside and cry "because she looked so beautiful."

The transformation had a different impact on Melissa. On the nights before a surgery, Melissa would say she wasn't going to be the same person the next day. After her surgeries, she refused to look in the mirror for days. Says Hardin, his eyes filling with tears, "She wouldn't look in the mirror because she wouldn't know who was going to be there."

Surgeries were planned around school vacations and summer break — typical for most children who have medical issues, so that they don't miss too much school. Because Melissa often had sutures, she had to avoid water and chemicals in pools, which meant no swimming. She had to be careful not to hit her head, so no Rollerblading or playing tag. No summer vacations at the beach. No trips to the Grand Canyon. No Disneyland, at least not until after the occasion of her 25th surgery, when Hardin took the entire family.

Since she was born, Melissa has enjoyed only two summer vacations and two Christmas holidays without a surgery, the first one in

2003. That year, when she was a freshman in college, she played — really played — outside in the snow for the first time. Late one evening, she and all her friends from her dormitory floor raided the school cafeteria for trays and set out in search of the perfect sledding hill. For the first time, she was inside the magical snow globe, not pressing her nose against its icy glass from the outside. She didn't have to watch while the kids rolled snowballs bigger and bigger until they had all the round parts for a snowman, left life-sized prints of angels in the snow, or had wicked snowball fights. She and her friends stayed out all night sledding and when she returned to her dorm room, her clothes were wet, her toes were freezing, and her face was as red as a holly berry. It was the best time ever.

ANY PARENT WHOSE CHILD has a craniofacial condition that requires numerous reconstructive surgeries always asks, "How much is too much? How do you know what's best? Whose decision is it? And how important is it to look 'normal'?"

Dealing with those issues is an art in itself, says Dr. Guyuron. One issue is taking care not to unintentionally communicate to children that something is very wrong with them and needs to be fixed. Sometimes, he says, parents are eager to have surgery for their children because they believe they themselves are to blame. Almost invariably, he says, that is not the case. So many birth anomalies simply happen by chance. Even when there's a genetic component to the anomaly, it certainly wasn't the parents' intention to pass it along to their child.

In most cases, the decision to have surgery is not left to the sole discretion of a parent. "Usually, it's the team that makes the decision. That team includes the surgeon, the parent or parents, the patient, and often, a child psychologist," says Dr. Guyuron. The team also may include a neurosurgeon, orthodontist, audiologist, otolaryngologist, and numerous other specialists, "just to make sure we're not myopic, we're not focusing on something that is in our area of expertise and ignoring the rest," he says. "As a surgeon leading the team, it is our responsibility to be cognizant of the patient, rather than the face, and focus on what goes on medically, physically, and emotionally, and bring all those factors into play to reach a prudent decision."

Doubting yourself and your decisions is so easy. The feeling is magnified when you're making decisions on behalf of someone else, the way Debbie had to for Melissa when she was younger.

"Nobody understands unless they walk in these shoes and have to put a child asleep so many times and wonder if they're going to come out of it better," she says. Any fear she felt about not doing the right thing for Melissa was offset by the tremendous confidence she had in Dr. Guyuron's expertise and his nurse Theresa's support. Theresa was always with Melissa, watching over her vigilantly, making sure she was okay. She was Melissa's guardian angel on earth and a comfort to Debbie.

The team helps parents to make decisions, but when children are old enough, usually in adolescence, they can begin to play a larger role. One major benefit is that whenever it is possible to give a child some choices about medical decisions — even surgeries — he or she will have a better surgical outcome and will heal better.

When children are too young to make decisions about having surgery, it's important to give them choices about surgery-related matters. Hospital child-life workers are crucial in this regard. They help children through the surgical process, giving them choices about how they might receive anesthesia or which hand they'd prefer for the IV. Although it might seem unimportant, those choices add up to calmer children and better results.

As she approached adolescence, Melissa was allowed to make decisions for herself. Dr. Guyuron would explain the reason for the procedure and allow her to have a say. He says she initially had some apprehension about certain procedures, but he recalls that "she really was a trooper," even through some of the major surgeries.

When Melissa turned 18, she, not her mother, became responsible for signing the consent forms for surgery. Dr. Guyuron, Melissa's mother, and the other team members had consulted with Melissa about procedures for years, and she knew her opinion mattered. Whether it was nodding "yes" to a procedure or articulating a concern about another, Melissa felt part of the decision-making process. But now she had to sign surgical consent forms, making what used to be a team decision feel like her decision alone. That privilege was clouded by a feeling of unwanted responsibility. "I knew it was something good, but I used to be able to blame it on my mother. Now I couldn't tell her it was her fault," she says, half-joking.

Often there are true functional benefits to craniofacial surgeries, such as improving a patient's ability to breathe, eat, speak, or see. The decision to undergo surgery in those instances seems easy. However, so many surgeries take their toll. When the fixes become more cosmetic in nature, or when a lack of function is tolerable, priorities may change.

Together, Debbie and Melissa made the decision not to have surgery on her ear when she was a teenager. Her ear canal is normal, but the nerves and muscles inside the ear are very different from those on the other side. Both women felt that Melissa had undergone so many surgeries already, and they were told that the ear surgery would be quite painful. Bone would have to be taken from her rib cage, and it just didn't seem worth it.

Melissa says that the last couple of surgeries — one on her nose to allow her to breathe out of both nostrils, and another on her jaw to extend and shape the bone and to place a chin implant — made a big difference in her appearance. More positive and confident than ever, Melissa is now at the point where she doesn't care so much what other people think. Her last surgery was July 5, 2004; a month later, she got good news from her orthodontist: She wouldn't need additional work. Good news, indeed.

THE INCIDENCE OF HEMIFACIAL microsomia is somewhere between one in 3,000 and one in 5,000. As with some other birth anomalies, the exact cause is unknown, although Dr. Guyuron says it might be caused by a blockage of one of the vessels that feeds blood to the segment of the face controlling the growth of the lower and upper jaw and cheekbone. The condition also may be inherited, although some experts disagree on this point.

"There is not a clear-cut inheritance pattern," says Dr. Anna Mitchell, a geneticist at the Center for Human Genetics at University Hospitals Case Medical Center in Cleveland, who is not surprised that there's some debate. The condition doesn't present with a typical inheritance pattern, and because a gene has not yet been isolated, whether hemifacial microsomia is inherited is open to interpretation, she explains.

Melissa's condition may have been a new onset, which means it was spontaneous, or it could have been inherited. It could have been the result of what's called multifactorial reasons, meaning alterations in more than one gene combined with environmental insults. Genetic evaluation and testing can offer some clues.

Genetic evaluation involves the collection of three types of information: personal medical history (starting from before birth, if possible), family history (ideally, at least three generations), and a physical examination. Multiple anomalies, such as dwarfism, extra digits, or congenital heart defects within a family, make it more likely that there is a genetic cause, particularly if the problems are related to each other. Anomalies that appear later in life are more likely to have an environmental component, Dr. Mitchell says.

If the results of the evaluation warrant further investigation, genetic testing can be performed. In Melissa's case, blood would be drawn in order to perform a karyotype, or chromosome analysis.

Dr. Mitchell explains it this way: A chromosome is to DNA what one encyclopedia is to a 22-volume set (humans have a total of 46 chromosomes in 22 numbered pairs, plus two sex chromosomes), and a gene is to a chromosome what a chapter is to a book. A karyotype is an organized method of arranging and viewing chromosomes to allow a researcher to identify an extra or missing chromosome, or to determine whether a chromosome has a piece broken off or if an extra piece attached itself to the chromosome.

A karyotype is performed by analyzing cells cultured from a blood sample under a microscope, to see whether any of the 46 chromosomes are irregular. "Chromosomes look like worms; they're stained to give them a banding pattern of white, black, and gray," says Dr. Mitchell. The cytogeneticist will check to see whether the chromosomes have the correct length and segmentation, and whether the banding pattern is correct.

If the chromosomes look normal, the family might leave with even more questions. "A normal karyotype does not mean that the condition is not genetic; it means it's not the result of a large rearrangement. If there is a genetic problem going on, it's something of a smaller scale than what we can resolve on a karyotype," says Dr. Mitchell. Using our earlier analogy, the analysis cannot tell whether every word on every page of the encyclopedia is spelled correctly. The technology is not yet that sophisticated.

"For some disorders, it's a single word spelled incorrectly on a page that's causing the problem," she says. "Make a misspelling in a different word and you get a completely different result."

When evaluating a patient for hemifacial microsomia, it is important to make sure that is the correct diagnosis. "There is overlap in the features of hemifacial microsomia and Treacher Collins syndrome," she explains. "The gene for Treacher Collins syndrome has been identified, so specific testing can be ordered for it."

Dr. Mitchell is careful about predicting risk, because much depends on individual circumstances and the results of genetic testing. Most children born with hemifacial microsomia have parents who are unaffected. The chance of those same parents having a second child with hemifacial microsomia is still slim — between 1 and 5 percent or so. If a parent has hemifacial microsomia, the chance of passing it on to a child is slightly higher, perhaps between 5 and 10 percent. Because a single gene has not been identified as the cause of the condition, researchers aren't sure that environmental factors don't play a role.

If a pregnant woman is at an increased risk of having a baby with hemifacial microsomia and wants to know whether her unborn baby is affected, Dr. Mitchell recommends a high-level or three-dimensional ultrasound study, which can pick up asymmetrical growth and facial anomalies. Having this information helps some people be better prepared if something is wrong.

Genetic testing is important to Debbie for those same reasons. If Melissa gets married someday and wants children of her own, she should know what the risks are, says Debbie. She'd also like her other children to know whether they could pass on a genetic mutation. Melissa promises she'll have the testing done.

FOR YEARS, DEBBIE NAVIGATED the medical, emotional, and physical demands of Melissa's condition alone. Her mother and sister were supportive, but they weren't equipped to support Debbie the way someone else in the same situation is. Like so many parents of children with disabilities, Debbie is grateful beyond words to the physicians and surgeons, but their role strictly involves the medical issues. They spend a few hours with patients, who are then put back into the public to fend for themselves, says Debbie.

"We need information for the real world," she says, comfortable in speaking on behalf of all parents in this kind of situation. For example, although Melissa was born with an eyelid, eyebrow, and eyelashes on her right side, she eventually lost all of them. Infection stole her eyelid and her eyelashes, and she lost her eyebrow from continually ripping off ocular eye patches, which were held fast to her face with strong adhesives.

"Dr. Guyuron thought that Melissa would do well if she could get eyelashes," says Debbie. So after "hours of phone calls" to various stores and finally a hospital burn center, she was referred to a local organization called Wigs for Kids. Although the staff was unable to help Melissa with new eyelashes, they did remove a section of her hairline that had grown into the area of her right eyebrow, and they suggested that she consider a permanent tattoo to replace her missing eyebrow. Melissa did get an eyebrow tattoo, and she keeps her hairline in check with occasional electrolysis treatments.

Despite all her surgeries and the physical pain afterward, Melissa says that she struggles most with the way people treat her: the staring and the comments. She feels safe at school and at home, but going out in public is demanding.

"I wish parents would educate their children that we're not all the same. I wish parents would tell children what's wrong and not just tell them not to stare," Melissa says, advocating for education rather than avoidance. In response to staring, Melissa usually just gives a little smile and walks away. But sometimes it's a challenge, and with a fair dose of sarcasm in her voice, she responds by asking, "Can I help you?"

THE LATE FRANCES COOKE MACGREGOR, an expert on the psychological effects of having a facial difference, found that people with facial differences use a number of strategies to cope in what she called a hostile environment. Staring is commonplace. Some people cope by simply pretending that they don't notice they're being stared at. Others cope by staring right back or by making a harsh comment. Still others just look away or move out of the person's line of sight.

Some hide, becoming veritable hermits. Others spend extraordinary energy compensating for their physical difference by being terribly interesting, witty, or positive. But to have to compensate for the benefit of others can become tiring quickly. One imagines a person with a facial difference asking, "Why must I compensate because my appearance doesn't meet your expectations? If you cannot accept me the way I am, why not at least compensate for your behavior toward me?"

Macgregor wrote that developing coping skills was no guarantee of a better or easier life. To the contrary, "The psychological costs of daily affronts, effort, and emotional strain are more often disproportionate to the social gains."

When we see someone who looks markedly different from any other person we've seen before, we're inclined to stare, at least for a few moments. It's as if our brains need extra visual information to understand what we're seeing. When we're met with a face, or any object, that looks so different from its archetype, we tend to take long looks.

So why is being stared at so unnerving? In the grand scheme of things, staring seems like a petty offense, certainly not as painful as a physical attack or even a verbal assault. When we stare at people, though, particularly people with a visible difference, we're sending messages to them that are uninvited. Whether we mean to or not, in their minds we're saying, "I see that you're different. I don't understand why you look that way. Your appearance puzzles or frightens me. There, but for the grace of God, go I."

People who are on the receiving end of stares will tell you that they feel like a target. In folklore, and still today in some cultures, a stare is the equivalent of giving someone the evil eye — a vicious curse that may be tempered only by wearing an amulet or a red string around the wrist. In the animal world, particularly in primates and dogs, staring is a way of asserting dominance. Predators stare down their prey before they attack and kill. From the earliest of times, staring has been an unwelcome advance.

All of us have been stared at on one occasion or another. Perhaps it was because our hair dye was past its expiration date and turned our hair the color of bile. Or perhaps it was because we dressed in the dark and showed up for an event with two different-colored socks. Whatever the reason, we were uncomfortable because we knew that our appearance was out of the norm. We weren't following the accepted social guidelines, and we stood out for all the wrong reasons. Now imagine feeling like that all the time.

Rosemarie Garland-Thomson is an associate professor of Women's Studies and director of graduate studies at Emory University in Atlanta. An expert in disability studies in the humanities and in women's studies, she recently wrote a book about staring.

"Staring is the human response to the visually novel," she says, adding that legibility or visual obviousness has a lot to do with staring behavior. For example, if you see a bald woman who looks as if she may be going through chemotherapy, you're less likely to stare, because you recognize her difference. The same is true with someone in a wheelchair or someone with a cast on his leg. These people have a particular look that is immediately identifiable. If you see young people walking down the street with brightly colored dyed hair and facial piercings and tattoos, you understand that they're part of a counterculture. However, Dr. Garland-Thomson explains, if you walk into a coffee shop and spot someone whose nose is missing, you're likely to stare because you don't understand what it means.

Your face is one of the few body parts that you cannot see without looking in a mirror. When you present yourself, you're not thinking about your long nose, your crooked teeth, or the scar that runs the length of your face. In other words, you're not fixated on that which you cannot see. You present yourself in the appropriate context of the situation, bringing forth your knowledge, skill, compassion, or humor. In a sense, you present yourself from the inside out, with your personality dominating. Usually, your physical self is an afterthought. However, if you have a facial difference and you're met with stares, you suddenly become keenly aware of your physical self, and your confidence in your nonphysical self is interrupted. The magic of the moment is gone.

Being stared at is so objectionable, says Dr. Garland-Thomson, because it is a reminder that "to someone else you are anomalous, scary, objectionable, or one of the many different things that staring means; whereas to you, you're just trying to get through your day. In modernity, one of the situations is that there is a tremendous standardization of the human body and of human life. For example, really in this culture we all dress alike, we all look alike — and there's a great deal of pressure to look alike. One of the privileges of normalcy in modernity is not being noticeable, not being stared at, not being seen."

The term used to define that type of anonymity is civil inattention, coined by the late sociologist and author Erving Goffman. In *Behavior in Public Places*, Goffman explains civil inattention as "enough visual notice to demonstrate that one appreciates that the other is present, while at the next moment withdrawing one's attention from him so as to express that he does not constitute a target of special curiosity or design." In other words, a cursory, civilized look to acknowledge someone else's presence, but certainly nothing more. Thus, civil inattention is what we offer people when we step into an elevator, for example, or when we take a seat next to them in the theater.

"That's what you lose, especially when you have any kind of facial difference," Dr. Garland-Thomson says.

There is comfort in not being in the spotlight, especially when the spotlight is focused on a difference that is linked with shame or embarrassment. It may be harder for those who were not born with a difference. "People move from one category to another. For example, someone who is in a car accident and sustains a permanent facial difference moves from civil inattention or visual anonymity into a space of visual attention. That's a huge change in your social status and your way of relating to people," she says.

Once people with facial differences become visually familiar to others, such as neighbors, classmates, or co-workers, they are much less likely to be stared at by those groups. Of course, this doesn't mean they wouldn't be stigmatized in other ways, says Dr. Garland-Thomson.

Although staring is inherent, she says, any sophisticated thinker knows that nature and culture are not in opposition. In other words, although staring may be biologically grounded, to stare at someone who is different is rude and improper. We must temper our biological urges with common courtesy and common sense.

The motto of Let's Face It, an information and support network for people with facial differences, offers excellent advice to those who are not facially different and who are tempted to stare at someone who is: To support people with a facial difference, look them in the eyes and smile at them.

Recently, Melissa and her sister, Kim, went for coffee together. Kim was wearing lime-green pants and a pair of hot pink shoes. As they were leaving the coffee shop, Melissa turned to her sister and said, "That was nice for a change: People were staring at you and not me!"

IN MATTERS OF DISABILITY or difference, familiarity breeds acceptance. From the time Melissa was born, her mother, sister, and brother surrounded her and lifted her. They never told her she couldn't do anything and never treated her as though she was different.

"We didn't give her an inch," says Tom, who is in his early thirties.

Because of that, Melissa grew up confident and capable. Despite the fact that she has a slight deficit in cognitive function, with difficulty in adding and subtracting (but, she's proud to say, she is a whiz at multiplication and division) and with short-term memory skills, Melissa was a good student and active in sports, playing soccer and taking gymnastics and ice-skating lessons. She also played softball. Her coaches worked with her so that she could hit the ball, and one year she won the outstanding player award.

"When I look at her, I don't see her difference," says Kim, who is two years older than Melissa. "Sometimes I even forget Mel is different."

To Melissa, that's a good thing, except when she can't hear what they're saying. Her family members forget that she can't hear out of her right ear, and they sometimes walk and talk on her right side without thinking. When Melissa turned 21, Kim and Tom took her to a nightclub. The club was packed with people, and the music was loud. Tom hollered something in Melissa's right ear, to which she replied, "What?" As he leaned closer to repeat it, Melissa's boyfriend intervened and yelled to Tom, "Other ear!"

Tom just shakes his head and laughs. "That's part of not holding her back," he says.

The acceptance through familiarity extended to school as well. Melissa was schooled in the same district from kindergarten through high school. Growing up with the same group of kids helped her to avoid being a target of teasing. Melissa's classmates were always kind to her. She wasn't picked on the way so many other children are — even "normal" ones. Even so, each year before school began, Debbie, and later Darrell Hardin also, would meet with Melissa's new teachers and explain her condition.

"We would explain to the children that she may look different, but she's still the same as they are, with her feelings and wanting to play," says Debbie. The teacher would explain Melissa's condition the first day and answer questions and concerns from the children. This way, if there was a problem, the teacher could deal with it right away. "I think that was the biggest key to her not encountering any problems."

DEBBIE TAUGHT MELISSA to walk with her head held high, because a parent can protect a child for only so long. At some point the child becomes an adult, and that adult has to walk on her own, says Debbie. Preparing Melissa to go to college — and preparing herself to let Melissa go — was a big step in that direction. But it wasn't done without a lot of effort.

"Society wants people to fit in and be productive, but there are so many obstacles," says Debbie. "There are programs available, but so many people don't know about them."

One of those programs is offered by the Ohio Bureau of Vocational Rehabilitation. By chance, Melissa's high school counselor directed the family to the Ohio BVR, where young adults with special needs or circumstances are prepared to survive and thrive in the real world. The BVR helps those who want to attend college make thoughtful decisions, connecting them with resources and helping them decide on a career based on their skills and interests. After meeting with BVR staff and being evaluated, Melissa was offered financial aid for college.

"For the first two years, the BVR paid her full tuition and books," says Debbie. However, because of state budget cuts, the program paid only a portion of Melissa's tuition for her junior year. She and her mother had to make up the difference, as well as pay for her books. Still, the BVR has been a big financial help.

Today, Melissa is a graduate of Kent State University, with the goal of being an intervention specialist for special-education kids. She's planning to work with children with mild to moderate attention-deficit disorder or slight memory loss.

"I'll help out in the classroom or help kids one-on-one to catch up or connect with things they missed in class. I want to give back to children who need extra help like I did," she says.

DURING A SUMMER BREAK while still in college, Melissa worked at a tooling shop, performing data entry. The shop is owned by a family friend who has known Melissa since she was a baby. The prior summer, she'd applied in person for jobs at several places, from retail stores to tanning salons, but she never got a call for an interview. She thinks it's because of how she looks. "No one ever called back," she says. It didn't take long for her to feel like giving up.

Her brother has several friends who've had a tough time finding a job recently. But unlike Melissa, he says, they won't feel that the rejection had anything to do with their appearance. For Melissa, every rejection will raise a question in her mind. Every rebuff, every turn of the cheek, every unreturned telephone call is evidence that someone thinks she's not acceptable.

In 1992, Title I of the Americans with Disabilities Act of 1990 took effect, the simplified intent of which is that employers with 15 or more employees cannot discriminate against qualified people with disabilities in matters of hiring, firing, compensation, and advancement. People with facial differences can be protected under Title I, but lawsuits brought under the act are notoriously difficult to win on behalf of the disabled person.

Arlene S. Kanter is a professor of law and co-director of the Center on Human Policy, Law, and Disability Studies at Syracuse University in New York, where she's been teaching disability discrimination law since 1990. "All cases under Title I are tough to win," she says, adding that many cases settle out of court, which may mean that one or both of the parties viewed their case as weak or, for other reasons, the parties simply preferred not to go to trial. Of those cases that do go to trial and the plaintiff wins, many are reversed on appeal, she says.

To be covered under the ADA, a qualified person must have a physical or mental impairment that substantially limits a major life activity, have a record of such impairment, or be regarded as having such an impairment. To be considered qualified, the person with a disability must be able to perform the essential functions of the job with or without reasonable accommodation, which brings up the question of what is reasonable accommodation. This is where the view gets cloudy. Reasonable accommodation is just that, and it remains so until it imposes "undue hardship" on the employer, taking into consideration the employer's "size, financial resources, and the nature and structure of its operation." Reasonable accommodation may be allowing a qualified employee to start work at 9:30 A.M. rather than 9 A.M. because the employee must rely on special transportation to get to work; it may be installing wheelchair ramps at all entrances; or it may be providing training materials in audio as well as in written format.

Title I tries to protect disabled individuals in the job application process, to the extent that a potential employer may not ask about the "existence, nature or severity" of a disability, only ability to perform the job functions. Still, if a disability is highly visible, such as a facial difference, there's little need on the part of the employer to ask about it. If a job offer isn't extended, the applicant may assume, rightly or wrongly, that it was because of the difference.

"It's hard to get into the mindset of the discriminator," says Kanter, which is why Title I cases against employers are so difficult to prove. The human resources manager conducting the interview may have felt the applicant didn't have the necessary skills to perform the job or the manager may have been thinking, "There's no way I'm hiring this person; she'll be a distraction to everyone, including the customers." Unless, in a moment of unlikely candor, the manager verbalizes the true reason, it's impossible to guess what he or she was thinking.

Playing offense may be the best tactic. Kanter recommends bringing up the disability or difference and assuring the prospective employer that it would not affect job performance in any way. Although this tactic will not eliminate discrimination, it brings the issue to the fore so that, it is hoped, the employer can make an intelligent decision.

"It's not the challenge of the individual, but rather the attitudes of others that prevent qualified people with disabilities from getting jobs," says Kanter. At times, the law does a woeful job of offering protection to prevent discrimination, and it may offer even less to those who have been discriminated against already.

ALTHOUGH DEBBIE DOESN'T blame herself for what happened to Melissa, knowing she didn't do anything wrong, she still wonders why Melissa was born with this condition. "I see young parents on drugs and they have normal kids. I'll question that till the day I die."

When Melissa was born, her mother wondered what kind of life she might have. In the hours after giving birth, Debbie wondered whether Melissa's condition was so serious that she'd have to fight for her life. If she survived, what would she have to fight for later? Would she have to fight for an education? A job? Acceptance?

But little prizefighter that she is, Melissa bounds into the ring every time. She keeps her feet moving and her eye on her target. The only thing she doesn't do is keep her head down. She holds it high, the way her mother taught her.

CHAPTER 7

the viking

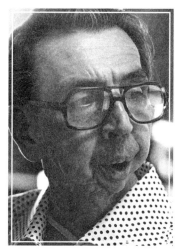

Jack Moyer

Do you ever watch the setting sun and dream of
things that you might have done?

—Perry Como, "When You Come
to the End of the Day"

JACK MOYER'S CANCER began as a lesion on the floor of his mouth, just below his tongue. It was 1972, and standard of care was to kill the cancer using what's called combined therapy: chemotherapy and radiation. Jack underwent a few weeks of chemotherapy. He then underwent radiation therapy to each side of his face and directly into his mouth, under his tongue, using a device shaped like a party hat. For weeks, his face and mouth were bombarded with radiant energy waves.

At that time, radiation therapy was a lot like carpet bombing. As careful as physicians were not to annihilate healthy tissue around a cancerous lesion, they were slaves to the limits of technology. There was no such thing as today's targeted radiation therapy. In Jack's case, the radiation ravaged his face like a wildfire, charring the skin to a shiny black and destroying everything in its path, including the cancer.

After Jack's treatments were over, the necrotic (dead) skin sloughed off, exposing new flesh that was hairless and spongy to the touch. The radiation destroyed not only the skin and tissue on his face but also the bone underneath. Several months after the radiation treatments were over, Jack had surgery to remove chunks of necrotic bone from his jaw, mainly his chin. At that time, a section of flesh along his lower left jawline tore open on its own, leaving a hole the size of a silver dollar.

Jack's physician told him that radiation acts differently with different people. "Well, personally speaking," Jack later wrote in his journal, "my reaction has been absolutely disastrous."

The wound leaked constantly, leaving a stain of whatever Jack had been eating or drinking on the bandage. His surgeon attempted to graft skin from various parts of his body to repair the wound several times, all without success. The surgeon also attempted several flap surgeries, using skin from Jack's neck and shoulder to fix the hole along his jawline. For the most part, the flap surgeries were unsuccessful and only resulted in leaving Jack's neck and shoulder disfigured. A few times, the tissue connected to his jawline turned black because it had died, and it had to be trimmed and reattached.

At one point, the hole in Jack's face healed after having been open for more than two years. He was thrilled. He wrote in his journal that the healing was monumental, calling the incision line "a beautiful sight" and adding, with his usual bit of good humor, "Look Ma, no holes." Only one other time in eight years did the wound along his jawline heal, giving Jack some respite, but the success was short-lived. His skin simply was too badly damaged to maintain healing.

BEFORE HIS CANCER, Jack was a very good-looking man, confident and charming. His face was framed by dark hair, which gave his dark brown eyes a certain intensity. He was athletic and sported a devilish grin that belied his gentle character. After his cancer and the ferocious firestorm of radiation, his appearance changed dramatically. The loss of his lower jaw caused his chin to look as though it had sunk into his neck. The open wound on the left side of his face, a nuisance he could never get used to, remained raw, and his skin turned thick and mushy.

Jack wrote about his disfigurement in his journal, noting that he now had the type of face that people in a crowd look at twice, "to make sure what they saw the first time is actually there." Yet he also wrote that he was surprised he didn't look worse because of all the surgeries he'd endured.

Jack's medical odyssey of the absurd kept getting more bizarre. When he developed a hole on the floor of his mouth, his surgeon attempted to repair it with a skin graft, using tissue from Jack's neck. Unlike so many of his other skin grafts, this particular one took. The only problem was that the skin on his neck was hair-growing tissue, so Jack ended up with hair growing beneath his tongue, a kind of inside-out beard. The hair was a constant, terrible irritation. When the hairs grew long and became a nuisance, he had them plucked out, ignoring his surgeon's curious advice to shave the floor of his mouth.

In the meantime, Jack was losing more and more of his lower jaw, along with many perfectly good teeth. The extensive grafts using bone from his hips and the microsurgery to minimize the continuing damage to his jaw failed.

Every attempt to patch his face and jaw seemed only to make matters worse. Finally, Jack, his surgeons, and his family had to accept that nothing more could be done. His skin, tissue, and bone were too badly damaged from the radiation. His face, terribly disfigured, was a wasteland where nothing could grow.

"I look like a freak to me," Jack wrote in his journal, "but not in the eyes of those who love me; and surely that has to be the most important thing. Love is still very dear, and each day I'm alive I thank God for that gift."

Eventually the cancer reappeared, seizing his throat. In a major surgical procedure, Jack lost part of his larynx and required a tracheotomy and feed tube. For the man who loved to laugh and sing, speech was now close to impossible, and eating wasn't much of an option.

"My aspirations are not as great as they used to be," Jack wrote. "My driving desire now is to be fitted with teeth and have my upper teeth either realigned or replaced and be able to bite a sandwich and chew, like normal people. I am a dreamer, but I am also a realist. This may never happen—if it doesn't, so what? I am still able to breathe in and out, and that simple function is a tremendous function."

Later, it became obvious that he wouldn't be able to swallow and that his only wish—to enjoy a simple hamburger on a bun with a slice of onion—would not be granted. Jack struggled to keep looking forward.

The inability to eat is a villain to which many people who have had oral cancer or numerous jaw surgeries can attest. Gone is the joy of eating a hot dog slathered in ketchup, mustard, and onions at the ballgame. Gone is the delight of letting a homemade chocolate brownie, still warm from the oven, melt in your mouth. Gone is the pleasure of patting a full belly and wiping an errant crumb from your lip. The joy of eating, so basic to our physical and emotional needs, is replaced with blended meals sipped through a straw or poured directly into a feed tube.

Still, like a lion in winter, Jack accepted the reality of not eating again with grace and humor. Bothered by television commercials that flaunted inch-thick steaks and steaming bowls of chili, he joked that he should embark on a personal crusade to convince the advertisers to "cut that out."

Jack Moyer underwent 63 surgeries in the eight years before he died in 1980. He was 58 years old.

DESPITE WHAT JACK MUST have been going through emotionally, to family, friends, and physicians, he was the Viking.

"I remember him going into surgery, being wheeled through the ward. He'd taken his surgical cap and fashioned it like a beret, cocked to the side, and he flashed the victory sign. He looked like Patton going open-eyed into the battle," recalls Jeff, who was 23 when his father's medical odyssey began.

Vikings put their own to death by making them jump into a pit of hungry wolves, armed only with their own sword. Death, of course, was unavoidable for the condemned warrior, but before being eaten, he could slay as many wolves as his courage and strength would allow.

"He was a Viking in the wolf pit, killing the wolves," says Jeff. "He fought. He never gave up."

At one point, his surgeon asked whether he wanted to stop treatment. Jack was just gearing up for a bone graft to replace bone he'd lost in his chin. "Let's go," he said. "I want all there is, and I'm ready to go after it." He wasn't about to strike the flag.

Although Jack didn't have the kind of counseling support we have today, he had faith that he didn't have more burdens than he could bear. "He kept looking for meaning and purpose, and, on some level, I think he knew that people admired how he handled adversity," says Jeff.

Despite challenges that would have brought others to their knees,

Jack treasured every day. Just prior to one of the last surgeries to try and rebuild his jaw, he talked about the tremendous pain in his mouth. He hoped the pain wouldn't become more than he could bear because the surgery was still five weeks away. He wrote, "You see, I don't want to wish my life away by hoping that the time goes by in a hurry."

Jack's surgeon and entire medical staff marveled at his resilience and perseverance. His surgeon said that he couldn't help getting personally involved with Jack and his family — probably, Jack suspected, because of all the procedures he'd performed on him in such a short period. Most patients would have given up, Jack wrote, "but this cookie isn't about to."

THE MIDDLE OF THREE children, Jeff is an advocate for all people with disabilities, probably because of his father's illness, his younger brother's severe cognitive disability, and his own disability: He's been blind since he was a young adult. Today Jeff is a musician, songwriter, and speaker. Among other things, he compiled an audio documentary examining life in pre-1990 state institutions for people with cognitive disabilities, and he created a musical and discussion guide on teasing and violence for elementary and middle school children.

Jeff says it would have been easy for outsiders to look at his father and think, "My God, what a horrible life!" The treatment for his disease destroyed his face, he couldn't work to support his family, one of his sons was slowly losing his vision, and his other son had been institutionalized.

"One of the things that happens to most of us when we experience loss is it opens our compassion to others. It opens our hearts," says Jeff, who grew up in Cleveland and still lives there today. "We've all experienced loss; it's a common denominator in our humanity. The attitudinal barrier becomes reduced only when we understand the true nature of loss. Then we can see each other as equals."

The challenge is that we're not good at dealing with loss and grief, and there's loss associated with any significant difference, says Jeff. In addition, our culture teaches us not to get close to others. So if we're faced with someone who looks different, and our first reaction is to avoid the person, we've created another barrier, another level of disconnectedness between ourselves and that person.

"When we take this holistic view of people with differences, we are not afraid to say to them, 'Excuse me, do you mind if I ask you what happened?' Then we understand and don't focus on it. Once they've told you what happened and you can express your compassion, then it's out of the way and you can talk about other things. If we're afraid, then we feel that it would be uncomfortable for them to talk about it," Jeff says.

If we are uncomfortable or afraid of a person because of his appearance, we cannot discover his stories or learn about his journey. Then the loss is shared by both of us.

David Roche, a humorist and speaker from Mill Valley, California, opens his speaking engagements by asking the entire audience to ask in unison, "What happened to your face?" David was born with an extensive cavernous hemangioma, which is a benign tumor made up of blood vessels, on the left side of his face and neck. Like Jack, he also endured over-radiation to treat his condition. By getting the question out of the way, David clears the air so that his audience can begin to see him as he sees himself, as a whole person. By acknowledging and accepting his flaws, he has made himself whole. That, he says, is the "core spiritual growth experience, an essential step in developing emotional maturity for all people, disabled and otherwise."

People have a difficult time seeing a disability as a normal attribute of a person's wholeness. "Disability does not create a unique psychology, a different human being. If I see you and treat you as whole, I can learn something. And it cuts both ways. Everyone benefits. This is recognition of our true unity," says Jeff. For example, he explains, if you see someone with a facial difference, your reaction shouldn't be, "My God, how do you leave home looking like that?" The reaction should be "There's a whole person in there."

A person with a disability is still a whole person with certain inalienable rights and the ability to achieve his or her own potential, based on the willingness to apply talents, skills, and abilities, explains Jeff. "We must challenge ourselves to move through our discomfort, move toward seeing someone with a disability as an equal. We need to recognize that person has a range of emotions that are just like our own," he says.

"If I look at you and my initial reaction is repulsion or fear, I'm inclined to back away," says Jeff. "When we avoid people who are different from us, we make them feel isolated and alone."

Jeff tells the story about a group of friends sitting around talking one evening. One of the men had a severe speech impairment, and Jeff could understand only a fraction of what he was trying to say. "I was afraid to ask him to repeat himself, so I found myself avoiding him. I'm guilty of it, too," he admits.

"What we've done with disability in our culture is set up a paradigm that means one of two things: One, you can do nothing, or two, the disability means nothing," says Jeff. With respect to the first, Jeff says that 92 percent of people admire those with a disability "just for showing up." This attitude of admiration, as he calls it, is bestowed on people with disabilities just for doing ordinary tasks because the overwhelming image of disability is helplessness.

Jeff will call a cab when he needs to go somewhere alone. He's perfectly adept at getting in and out of cars, but on one particular day, as he crawled inside, the cabdriver patted him on the back and gave him an "atta boy!" Years ago this experience would have made Jeff feel humiliated, but because he's attained self-acceptance, he's unaffected by those comments and attitudes.

"The vast majority of people are acting out of good intentions," he says. Still, the take-home message is, "Admire my talent, not my ordinary activities!"

With respect to a person's disability meaning nothing, Jeff gives the example of the late actor Christopher Reeve, who everybody knew as Superman. "We want to believe that people with disabilities can do anything, like climb Mount Everest even though they're blind. We want to believe that people with disabilities can achieve anything, and we look to the few who do and feel good. But most don't achieve super-human goals; they live ordinary lives," he says.

Most people with challenges can overcome them, and their challenges don't occupy the centerpiece of their life, says Jeff. However, an exception may be those people with facial differences.

"The nature of facial disfigurement is a difference that's devalued. A devalued difference is deviant, and that's how those with facial differences are often seen. I can't think of one example of anyone with facial disfigurement that is lifted up as a role model or superhuman exemplar," says Jeff. "Every encounter is a fresh reminder that people see you as a different person. Life goes on, but you become one-dimensional in other people's eyes."

For people with facial differences, there's a tremendous amount of insecurity when they're in social situations because they don't know how people are going to react to them. Thus, at the outset, people with facial differences experience a barrier to social interaction.

Renowned social scientist Frances Cooke Macgregor wrote extensively about people with facial differences and social interactions. In studies of hundreds of people, she found that the reactions of strangers were far more hurtful than any emotional pain they felt when they looked at themselves in the mirror.

These painful encounters took place when traveling to work or school, shopping, entering and eating in a restaurant, walking along the street, or standing in line. In other words, in everyday living.

One day, Jack was in his brother's office when he recognized an old friend in the waiting room. He and this man had been friends for nearly 30 years; Jack had even served as the best man in his friend's wedding. Jack wanted to shout hello, but his voice was gone by then. He attempted to make eye contact, but the man just looked away. Jack's brother entered the waiting room and saw that the two old friends were not speaking. He approached the man and said, "Ed, you remember my brother, Jack," to which Ed replied, "No, I don't believe we have met."

Jack was unsettled by that encounter, but it helped him realize how different he looked. "I guess I am still looking at life through the same pair of eyes as before I found a spot under my tongue. The eyes see as before, but what people see when they look at me is someone different," he wrote.

There are lessons to be learned from those who have journeyed where we have not gone and where we wouldn't choose to go. Jeff insists that we should be willing to accept people who are different, treat people with respect, and be open to the lessons they can teach. "The older I get, the more I realize the incredible value and meaning of my father's life," he says.

After the attempt at rebuilding his jaw failed, Jack was sorely disappointed. It was the surgery he had looked forward to most, because he had hoped it would allow him to be able to eat again. That loss, coupled with the fact that his cancer returned, shook him profoundly, and he turned his thoughts toward what he might have to offer others.

"Experience is a tremendous teacher, and it seems a shame that it takes sorrow to have to be the predecessor for knowledge," he wrote. "In my lifetime I have learned a lot about a lot of things, and it seems that's about all I have to leave to anyone. First, love one another very deeply, and don't be ashamed to express your love openly and often. Also, enjoy one another, and guard zealously your time together so as to enjoy it to the fullest extent."

BORN JOHN W. MOYER, known as Smiling Jack in his youth, Jack was a fun-loving man. He met his wife, Louise, in elementary school.

They began dating in high school and were married shortly after graduating. With a couple of years of medical school under his belt, Jack joined the U.S. Navy. He served in the Pacific theater during World War II, working in a receiving hospital for wounded soldiers and doing everything from performing triage to running a psychiatric ward.

Jeff remembers his father telling him a story about the hospital's lack of decent bandages. Tired of making do, Jack organized the hospital staff to contribute one-third of their pay to purchase quality supplies. To him, it wasn't enough that the wounded soldiers might be happy simply to be alive, the soldiers deserved the best care and supplies money could buy.

After his stint in the service, Jack became an industrial salesman in the steel industry. Not long before he was diagnosed with cancer, the steel industry fell into a slump and he lost his job. The prospects of finding a similar job looked grim. For his father's birthday and to give him something to do between jobs, Jeff bought him a model kit of a wooden sailing ship.

"It sat under the bed for six months," says Jeff. But then Jack retrieved the model from beneath the bed to take a closer look. During the course of his illness, he built one ship after another, finding therapy in building something with his hands. One year, Jack won six ribbons for his ships at a local county fair, and his surgeon commissioned him to build a model of Nova Scotia's most famous tall ship, the Bluenose schooner.

To craft a simple ship — say, a 20-inch schooner — would take Jack six weeks, working 12 hours a day. A more complex ship, such as the USS *Constitution*, would take up to six months. The detail, precision, and accuracy of his craftsmanship were a testament to his willpower and desire to leave something beautiful behind. "He wanted his life to matter," says Jeff.

Hunched over a small table with an unfolded schematic, a bottle of glue, and hundreds of pieces of basswood that he had meticulously cut to prescribed dimensions, Jack would build his ships. One by one, he'd pick up each piece and glue it into place with surgical skill. Slowly the mound of basswood pieces would grow smaller, and the ship's form would take shape, rising into view like a phantom ship — the *Flying Dutchman* sailing out of the eye of a storm.

Taking a ball of ropelike string, Jack would methodically construct the running rigging, weaving the fibers through the cotton sailcloth that he'd cut himself, tying them off, and clipping the long ends. He'd add brass stanchions and cannons to the deck, string the life preservers, and run the flags. Using careful brushstrokes, he'd add color to the hull or cabin.

From a jumble of pieces and parts, Jack made each ship whole, with nothing left over and nothing missing. The ships were masterpieces, probably seaworthy. Working well into the night, Jack must have wondered why his surgeons couldn't do the same for him.

During the hours Jack spent at the table, he was able to forget about the pain in his jaw, the uncertainty of his future, the next looming surgery and hospitalization, and the fact that he couldn't enjoy a hamburger. Jack's schooners, clippers, and tall ships took him to another place, surrounded by serene waters and open skies. When the wind caught the sails just right, the ships would slice through the water like a blade. Alone on one of his ships, Jack was comforted by the rhythmic sound of the water slapping the ship's hull. The clean smell of salt air filled his lungs. He'd sail for hours, always keeping an eye on the horizon for a glimpse of shore, a reminder of his family waiting for him at home.

AT ONE POINT BETWEEN surgeries, Jack was well enough to putter around in his workshop. Jeff wanted to take a photo of him working. At first, Jack resisted, but then he relented to make his son happy.

After the photo was developed, Jeff was eager to see it. He held it close, using a magnifying glass to see his father's face. His father had little jawbone by then, and his face was badly sunken on the left side. A tube of tissue ran from his neck to his chin, another attempt to repair the gaping wound along his jawline. Jeff was heartbroken by the image.

"I saw the anguish in his eyes and felt he didn't want the photo of himself disfigured because that would be what was remembered," Jeff says. Although he took the photograph as a way of honoring his father, he says he wishes he had been sensitive to his resistance. "What I didn't appreciate was that he was still experiencing his loss."

Jack's illness was a private test of endurance. "My father never had any psychological or social support for everything he went through. He never had a way to put his experience into context: no way to process his losses," says Jeff. "He lived with isolation that must have been so painful."

PART OF JEFF'S ADVOCACY work involves helping people gather the tools they need to cope and succeed so they don't have to endure their challenges alone. He feels that role models are vital, particularly for children with disabilities. "If a child has a facial disfigurement, connect them to someone like them," he says.

Not only are support groups a good starting place to find role models, but they also serve a crucial purpose for people with disabilities. Being among people with similar situations and stories creates a connection and a shared language. In a community of sameness, the disability becomes normal, says Jeff, and support groups offer a safe place to grieve openly, work out feelings, and come to terms with losses.

After Jack's death and until hers in 1995, Louise lived with an unexpressed sorrow, a deep sadness, because she didn't know how to grieve over the enormity of what she had lost. "My parents were of a generation that didn't benefit from our changing social norm about the requirement to process loss and seek psychological wellness," says Jeff.

Had she had the right kind of support and the vocabulary to talk about her loss, perhaps her remaining years would have been more peaceful. Although she was strong and resilient, Jeff says, his mother lived with a "quiet desperation that didn't need to be there." Today, we know better, he says. Because the human experience involves loss, we need to feel it, express it, and then release it. Only then do we achieve healing.

TOWARD THE END OF Jack's life, he developed lung cancer, which resulted in repeated bronchial infections. His lungs filled with fluid, and he had to be hospitalized. While he was lying in bed, something startled him, and he raised himself up on his elbows. Jeff reached for his father, holding him to take the weight off his elbows and ease him back down into the bed. At that moment, Jeff could see right into his father's eyes.

"He had a look of awe, of complete surrender. It was beautiful," Jeff recalls. And then Jack died.

Jeff carefully snaps a tape into a cassette player and turns up the sound. The tape is about 25 years old. Jack and Louise are singing their rendition of an old Perry Como song. You can almost see the couple beaming at each other as they sing; each has one arm around the other and each has a hand on the microphone. Harmonious and hopeful, they sing, their voices reflecting quiet resiliency in the face of illness and uncertainty. The Viking, who set out on an impossible journey, sang the words without regret: "Do you ever watch the setting sun and dream of things that you might have done?"

The USS *Constitution*, Jack's finest work, has its moorings in Jeff's home. The majestic ships he built are only part of his legacy. Although Jack said he would have done anything in his power to avoid having cancer, the disease allowed him to discover the love that was all around him. "I have the greatest wife a man could hope for, the finest children, and with all that, I am a very wealthy man," he wrote shortly before his death. "I am rich in things no one can buy — love, consideration, prayers, friendships — and I could have never realized it without something like a small touch of cancer."

Jack's spirit was buoyed by the love of his family. And when he finally set sail, he left peacefully, the way a man can when he's had a life well lived.

⊗

CHAPTER 8

i gotta be me

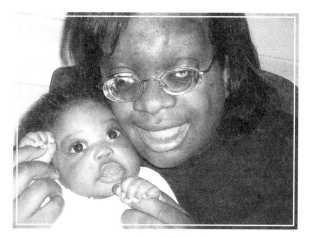

Latrea Wyche and baby Olivia

What lies behind us and what lies before us
are small matters compared to what lies within us.

—Ralph Waldo Emerson

WHEN THE FRONT DOOR opened, a bubbly four-year-old bounced right up to Donna Mance and asked, "Are you gonna be my new mommy?" Before Donna could answer, a slight girl standing at a distance caught her eye. Her small-framed body hugged the wall, and Donna noticed that she kept her head down. *That's Latrea,* she thought. She had been given some background on the two girls from the social worker who specialized in placing children in foster homes. Just a year earlier, Latrea and Ashley were removed from their mother's care. Donna had been told about the homes that rejected Latrea because her face was disfigured.

"I went there not really knowing how I was going to feel at that moment," says Donna, but she was drawn to Latrea. "I just couldn't see her being pushed aside. She seemed like a little lost puppy. I just wanted to reach out to her and let her know it was all right. Just wanted to protect her from the treatment she'd been used to receiving."

Donna understood that their current foster mother wanted to keep Ashley, Latrea's younger sister, but wanted Latrea removed. Thinking Latrea's condition might be contagious, the foster mother kept her away from the rest of the family, including the other foster kids. She wouldn't allow her to go near her baby or sit on certain furniture, including the chairs and couch in the living room.

The foster mother's biological daughter couldn't stand to look at Latrea. She said it made her sick to sit at the table with her, so Latrea was made to eat her meals alone or with Ashley. Because her foster mother couldn't stomach the thought of her eating off the same plates and drinking from the same cups as the rest of the family, Latrea had to eat from paper plates and use plastic forks, spoons, and knives — lesser-quality items, easy to toss aside. Usually, Latrea drank from paper cups, too, but sometimes she was allowed to have a plastic cup, one that was just for her.

When she was very young, Latrea would host tea parties for her stuffed animals. Everyone ate from the same dishes and drank from the same cups. It didn't matter that her teddy bear's ear was torn or her Cabbage Patch doll was dirty. Everyone was invited to the table.

While she lived in that house, Latrea floated like a voiceless ghost, moving softly from empty corner to empty corner. She crept around the perimeter of the house on tiny feet, careful not to step too heavily, make too loud a noise, or leave a footprint. Who would want to leave any part of herself there anyway?

Donna stepped inside the house. When the foster mother greeted her, all she could think was, *What kind of human being are you?*

ONE SUMMER DAY, the foster mother drove her daughter, Latrea, and Ashley to a nearby shopping mall — a real treat. Young girls love malls. They like to look at the clothing, the jewelry, and the other shoppers. But when they arrived, their foster mother told Latrea and Ashley to wait in the car.

"She didn't want to take my sister into the store and leave me in the car," says Latrea, "and she didn't want to take me in the store because she was embarrassed." The only option from her perspective was to leave both girls in the car.

That day was hot, and Latrea and her little sister sat in the car for several hours, waiting for their foster mother and her daughter to return. Even with the car windows open, the girls were sweltering. Latrea knew that she couldn't panic; that would just upset Ashley. *If I fall apart, she'll fall apart*, she thought. She knew she had to stay calm and occupy Ashley for as long as it took.

As frustrated as Latrea felt, she didn't believe running away was an option; how could she leave Ashley behind? Latrea was sure she had the street smarts to make it on her own, but she wasn't convinced she could take care of her sister. She couldn't jeopardize her sister's well-being; she couldn't jeopardize her life.

One morning before school, Latrea was left standing at the bus stop. She'd arrived too late and missed her bus. Ashley had already caught hers and was on her way to school. Rather than going back home, Latrea decided to walk to school. She needed something warmer than the pink windbreaker she was wearing, but she wasn't about to go home. She was determined to walk, and walk she did, for miles.

(A year earlier, Latrea's biological parents had been thrown out of the town house where they had been living. Her mother led her and Ashley out the door and past all their belongings piled on the curb. As they walked up the street, Latrea turned to see her father standing by the curb, guarding their things. But they kept walking, for hours and hours. "It got so bad, I had to put Ashley on my back. She didn't want to walk anymore," Latrea remembers. Several days later, they were still walking.)

The short way to school turned into the long way around. Sixteen hours later, the police picked her up. "Let's just say I was a long ways away from home," she says, laughing. Although Latrea was cold and tired, she was more determined to make a point. Running away was the only leverage she had with the social workers to get different foster-care placement. Only she knew the reality: She never would have left Ashley behind and she would not have brought her along. *Please, someone help us*, she thought.

Latrea's spirit was breaking. The child who loved to play on the monkey bars was tired all the time. The girl who beamed whenever she did a handstand now rarely smiled. Little feet that liked to run began to drag. Latrea felt her world getting smaller. She went for weeks at a time without saying a word, her mouth tasting like dust. "I could have rolled into a ball and disappeared," she says, "and nobody would have noticed."

That was when, like an angel, Donna came knocking. Because the county wanted to keep the sisters together, the social worker called Donna, who had been a foster parent for nine years at that point, taking in only special-needs children. She had four children of her own and would eventually adopt seven more. She took a ride out to the foster home where Latrea and Ashley were staying.

"Her sister could have easily been placed or adopted out because she had no handicap," says Donna. "But Latrea wasn't because of the features of her face. No one wanted to take her."

After treating the girls to dinner, Donna took them back to her home. Latrea immediately felt safe. The neighborhood was quiet. No gunshots or yelling. She imagined she could sleep safely there — in her own bedroom! — and she was certain no one would try to break into the house. The girls met Donna's two adopted boys, and Latrea realized that all the kids there had special needs. "I remember thinking either she's crazy or really nice!" she says. After a couple of visits, she and her sister moved in.

"I WAS TOLD THAT, at birth, they knew something was not particularly right about me," says Latrea. Her eyes slanted downward and were set wide apart, and the bridge of her nose was missing, causing her nose to look as if it had been smashed into her face. At first, everyone thought she might have had Down syndrome. Testing, however, would reveal that Latrea was born with a rare genetic condition called Pfeiffer's syndrome. She has Type I, which is the most common form and, unlike Type II and III cases, typically doesn't involve cognitive deficits.

The syndrome is characterized by premature fusion of the skull bones, called craniosynostosis, either at birth or early in childhood. Immediate medical care is often required; otherwise, brain growth may be stunted and other serious conditions can develop, such as cerebellar tonsillar herniation, in which part of the brain is squeezed into the spinal canal, and hydrocephalus, a buildup of fluid in the brain.

Pfeiffer's syndrome also is characterized by underdeveloped facial bones that don't grow far enough forward. Shallow eye sockets make the eyes appear to bulge. The mid-face area often is squished, giving the face a short, wide appearance and causing breathing problems. Children with Pfeiffer's syndrome typically have smaller nasal passages and occasionally a narrower trachea, or windpipe. At eight weeks, Latrea underwent cranial surgery to separate her fused skull bones, and she was given a tracheotomy so that she could breathe. She would need it until she was five.

Children with Pfeiffer's typically are hearing impaired and have poor vision. Latrea is no different. She has less than 50 percent hearing in her left ear and between 60 and 70 percent in her right ear, and there's no guarantee her hearing won't get worse. She's worn hearing aids since birth. She could also lose her remaining vision at any time.

The syndrome is an autosomal dominant disorder, which means that the chance of a child inheriting the disorder from his or her parents is 50 percent. Most cases of Pfeiffer's syndrome, including Latrea's, are the result of a spontaneous mutation — meaning that neither parent had the syndrome, but for some unknown reason, the combination of their genes resulted in a genetic mutation affecting their child. Pfeiffer's syndrome is related to Apert and Crouzon syndromes, two similar craniofacial disorders with autosomal dominant inheritance patterns.

Pfeiffer's is caused by a genetic mutation on chromosomes 8 and 10, areas that control fibroblast growth receptors. Dr. Anna Mitchell, a geneticist at the Center for Human Genetics at University Hospitals Case Medical Center in Cleveland, explains that fibroblasts are cells found in connective tissue, skin, and bone. When the fibroblast growth receptors are damaged, they cannot process growth messages correctly. Thus, babies with Pfeiffer's are born with problems resulting from facial and skull undergrowth or overgrowth, such as craniosynostosis. Still, geneticists can pinpoint the cause in only 70 to 80 percent of people with Pfeiffer's. This may mean that another gene, one that hasn't been identified yet, is involved in the syndrome, says Dr. Mitchell.

Knowing this is crucial to Latrea, who is married and expecting her first baby. "They told me there's a 50 percent chance my child will have it," she says.

If the mother or father has the syndrome and the mutation has been identified through genetic testing, amniocentesis can determine whether the baby has it, too. Latrea underwent genetic testing when she was a young girl, but she doesn't recall particulars of the results.

If neither parent has the syndrome, if an affected parent hasn't had genetic testing, or if the affected parent falls in that 20-to-30-percent group in which the mutation cannot be identified, a three-dimensional ultrasound may pick up facial and skull abnormalities, says Dr. Mitchell. So far, Latrea's ultrasound results show that the fetus looks okay, but there's really no way of knowing for sure until the baby is born.

"I'm excited and scared," says Latrea. "I know that all parents hope for the best and hope their children come out healthy, but I think I'm better prepared than most other parents. I have gone through it. If my child were to have it, I'd know what to do, what doctors to see, what help to get." Either way, her baby will be lucky.

WHEN LATREA WAS FIVE years old, she remembers going to Charlottesville, Virginia, for cranial surgery. The surgeon was an expert in treating children with Pfeiffer's syndrome. "I remember being really sad and wanting my dad to come with me. I was waving to him out the window as we drove by."

After the surgery, Latrea's mother told her husband that their daughter was on her deathbed so that he would come to the hospital. He was uneasy about being in hospitals. When he arrived, Latrea, who actually was recovering nicely, crawled up into his lap, and someone took their photograph. It was Christmas Day, 1985. That Polaroid is the only photo Latrea has of him.

LATREA SHOWED UP FOR her first day of kindergarten happily toting her book bag. Her eyeglasses had lenses almost as thick as glass-block windows, and she wore a helmet to protect her head. She still had a tracheotomy and couldn't speak very well. She took her suctioning machine to school so that she could clear her trachea throughout the day. It wouldn't be easy for Latrea to make friends.

She wasn't allowed to play outside during recess; the teachers were too worried that she'd hit her head and get hurt. While the other children tumbled out the school doors to play, she had to curl up on a blanket in the back of the classroom and take a nap. She could hear the sounds of laughter, feet chasing after balls, the smacks of jump ropes hitting the asphalt. Latrea, a tomboy at heart, had to lie on her blanket, imagining herself on a swing, being lifted higher and higher — above her classmates, above her teachers, high above the entire school. Then one day, the physical education teacher came into her classroom and announced to the teacher that Latrea could play outside. "It was the happiest day of my life!" she says. "You would've thought I'd never been outside before!"

But being able to play outside wasn't a panacea. She was still lonely. "We were playing ring-around-the-rosy or something that required holding hands. I wanted to play. Nobody wanted to hold my hand," she says.

Once, a girl held her hand and then wiped it on her shirt, fearing she would contract whatever it was Latrea had. Mainly, the kids felt sorry for her and avoided teasing her. It was an unwritten rule: We can't be her friend, but let's at least not make fun of her.

LATREA'S BIOLOGICAL MOTHER WAS a drug addict. Her father was an alcoholic. As time went by, more and more money was spent supporting habits and less was left for rent and food. The family moved from one apartment to another, sometimes leaving before the eviction notice could be taped to the door. Drug and alcohol addiction makes a peculiar prison. Many addicted persons won't think twice about sacrificing everything they have — their jobs, their lives, their own children — for a longer sentence. When Ashley was born, Latrea, then eight, was told the baby was her responsibility. It was her job to care for her baby sister, whose blood vessels pulsed with traces of crack cocaine.

Latrea did everything she could to give Ashley a stable home life. Although she was just a kid herself, she took on the role of parent to her sister. "I taught her how to read. I taught her how to ride a bike. I made sure she did her homework. I made sure she got on the bus to school. I made sure she got home safely." She pauses and adds, "Those were trying times."

DURING THOSE TIMES WHEN Latrea had no one, she held onto her faith, something she believes she was born with. "And I'll tell you, faith takes you a long way. I know I wouldn't be where I am right now if I didn't have my faith. The Bible says we're all put on this earth for a purpose. I thank God for the tragedy. I thank God for the mishaps. It was God's way of shaking me and molding me into the person I am. Some will make it over the hurdles, and some won't."

Latrea's father gave her up when she was about 14 years old. She was in Children's Hospital in Washington, D.C., when he showed up at her bedside. He told her, "I'm an alcoholic and I'm going to be an alcoholic to the day I die. I can't take care of you or give you what you need." And then he told her he'd signed away his parental rights.

"In a way, I respect him for that. He was honest. He didn't try to pretend. He said, 'My children shouldn't have to suffer because of me.'"

Considering all she's been through, Latrea should not have finished high school, much less gone to college, married a good man, and begun to establish a comfortable life. Latrea was left to rear her baby sister herself. She had complex medical issues that required major surgeries. She was insulted and taunted and ignored at school and in public. She moved from foster home to foster home and back to her biological mother again and again. When she was finally adopted, she was 16, almost a legal adult.

"You have to make up your mind that you're not going to let your situation dictate how you're going to be. You have to take your situation and turn it around and make it work for you," she says. Latrea faced more adversity before she was an adult than most people encounter in their entire lives. Perhaps it was the hard times that fueled her. Had it not been for having all the odds against her, perhaps she wouldn't have been so determined.

Each year, in elementary school, the fifth- and sixth-graders went on a camping trip for a few days. "I really wanted to go," she says. "I was determined I was going to go." The trouble was, she had no clean clothes — "none whatsoever," she says. Her mother kept promising to take her dirty laundry to the Laundromat, but the night before she was to leave for the trip, the pile of soiled clothing still lay on her bedroom floor. Latrea filled the bathtub with water and dish soap, washed her clothes, and then hung them on the line outside, thinking that by morning they would be dry. They weren't. Undeterred, she neatly folded her wet, cold pants, shirts, socks, and underclothes in her suitcase. "I was going camping!" she laughs.

When she got to school, her teacher was a little suspicious about what was in her suitcase. Maybe the outside was wet, or maybe the suitcase was heavier than it should have been. She insisted on looking inside and discovered the mound of wet clothing. Familiar with Latrea's home situation and being fond of her, the teacher wasn't going to leave her behind. With Latrea in tow, she went to the Laundromat. And Latrea went camping.

SEVEN MONTHS INTO HER pregnancy, Latrea heads to the emergency room because of pain. Her doctor puts her on complete bed rest. If the baby is born now, its lungs may not be developed well enough to allow it to survive. Some of the complications are because of Latrea's condition. Her body is tiny and frail. Carrying a child is a challenge, especially as the baby grows.

WHEN LATREA WAS A young girl, she noticed that people stared at her. Everywhere she went, people looked at her. She didn't understand why. As she got older, strangers made remarks or moved to another table if they happened to be sitting near her in a restaurant. One time, three men seated near her thought it was great fun to laugh at her. By this time she understood, and she lowered her chin to her chest.

"I went off!" says Donna, who told Latrea to raise her head. "What do you think you're looking at?" she growled at the three men.

"Ma'am, I don't mean no harm," one said.

"What do you mean, you don't mean no harm! She's a human being!"

At that point, Mr. Mance gave his wife a long look, so she didn't say anything else to the three men. "I probably said more than I should have," she laughs.

Incidents like that led to many long discussions about what "normal" looks like. Latrea would tell Donna, whom she calls Mom, that she wanted to be normal and her mother would reply that nobody's normal. "None of us is perfect. We all have some hang-ups or baggage that we travel with, be it on the outside or inside," says Donna. "She just had a hard time with society. When they looked at Latrea, they didn't see a sweet child; they just saw her outside appearance. I want people to see how beautiful she is. I wish they'd stop and give her a chance."

LATREA AND ASHLEY WERE returned to their biological mother several times before Donna was finally able to adopt them. Their mother would get the girls back for a while and then they'd be taken away again because she'd fail a random drug test. The girls were returned to their mother a couple of weeks before Christmas one year. On Christmas Eve, Donna brought their holiday gifts to their apartment. She remembers walking in and seeing that the girls didn't have a Christmas tree and didn't have any gifts. She put the gifts she'd brought on the floor.

The girls opened their presents, and Latrea was thrilled to receive her very first watch. It wasn't until she was nine or ten years old that she finally learned to tell time. She thought, *I got a watch, and I know how to use it!*

As Donna was leaving, she looked back at the apartment building and saw Latrea sitting in the front window, holding back the sheet that served as a curtain, watching her. Latrea's eyes followed Donna as she walked down the sidewalk, negotiating mounds of dirty snow to get to her car. She watched Donna hesitate beneath a flickering street lamp, then unlock the car. She watched her climb in and start the car, the sound of the motor fresh for just a moment, until it was swallowed by the din of sirens. She watched Donna for another minute while the car warmed up and then followed the path of the car as it pulled into the street, its plume of exhaust rising silently into the night.

Driving home, Donna could only pray that the girls knew she loved them and wanted them. Even to this day, when she recalls that evening, she says, "I don't even like thinking about it."

Within days, the girls were removed from their biological mother after a random drug test showed she was using drugs. Latrea and Ashley landed in the home of a church deacon and his wife. They kept the sisters in the corner from the time they arrived home from school until well past their bedtime. The girls weren't allowed to use the bathtub more than once a week and they were dressed in dirty clothes. It would take an entire year, but finally the school called Children's Services to alert them that the girls were being neglected. Latrea and Ashley were removed from that home and placed permanently with Donna.

TO BE ADOPTED, LATREA, then age 16, had to testify in court in front of her biological mother that she didn't want to live with her anymore. "I wouldn't wish that on anyone. It was the hardest thing I've ever had to do," she says.

She knew, though, that if she wanted an opportunity to have a stable life, she had to do it. "After being in the system so long, after living in poverty so long — I'm talking poverty, days without food, my mother selling anything she could get her hands on to get drugs — I knew this wasn't what my life was supposed to be," she says. "I always knew there was something better; I just had to get there. Whatever that better was, I had to find it. I'd always think, this is just a roadblock to where you need to be. I felt like I owed it to myself and my sister to create a stable life. It hurt me to my heart, but at the same time, I knew that it was the only way. If I had gone home with her, I wouldn't be what I am today."

By this time, Latrea had spent a lot of time with the Mances, and the chance to be adopted with her sister into the same home was golden. "That was the problem. Not too many people want to adopt older kids and sickly kids. They want babies and toddlers and 'normal' kids," says Latrea. "A lot of parents wanted Ashley, but they didn't want me."

Although many people told Latrea it was the right decision, she felt as though she had turned her back on the person who brought her into the world, and for the longest time she couldn't shake the image of her mother sitting in the courtroom. Her mother wore a light green suit that day and sat straight up in her chair. She looked as though she fit in, maybe could even have been a court reporter. She didn't say much. She just sat in that chair, her face like stone.

Latrea says, "To this day — and this was many, many moons ago — I can still close my eyes and see the look in her eyes."

ONE OF THE FIRST THINGS Donna did after Latrea moved in was to take her to the Children's Medical Center in Washington, D.C. A nursing assistant who worked with handicapped children for 24 years before retiring, Donna wanted to make sure Latrea received whatever medical treatment was necessary. For one thing, Latrea was missing her front teeth — they never came down — and her gums protruded. Also, her forehead and eyes drooped, giving her a woebegone look. Donna and Latrea spent the entire day at the hospital, meeting a team of specialists, including geneticists, dentists, plastic surgeons, and neurosurgeons, so that they could get a complete picture of what Latrea needed. At the end of the day, their plan was to fix the alignment of her mouth and fit her with dentures to replace her missing front teeth. The surgery would be her second of that kind; when she was seven or eight, her jaw had been broken and wired shut to bring it into alignment.

This second surgery would not only improve Latrea's appearance but also help eliminate the digestive problems she was having from chewing her food improperly. The team also recommended replacing missing bone in her skull using coralline hydroxyapatite, which comes from coral and is highly compatible with the body. Over the course of the next several years, Latrea would undergo several surgeries to align her jaw and fill in the spaces in her skull.

The next focus was academics. In the Mance household, the girls learned that education was a priority. "Nobody slides," says Donna. Latrea was terribly behind in school, so Donna started with the basics. She bought Latrea stacks of workbooks and spent hours helping her catch up. "She would get mad at me and my husband, thinking we were too hard on her," recalls Donna.

"She was an outcast in school, so I always told her to be smart," she says, adding that people only see you for what's on the outside; they don't know what you're capable of on the inside. Sure, it would take her longer to learn. She'd probably even need more time to take tests. Donna arranged an individual education plan for Latrea so that she would get the special services she needed.

The message to Latrea was clear, repeated over and over: You're not stupid, you're not ignorant, you're not dumb. But you are going to have to work twice as hard as everybody else. And you can do it; I know you can do it.

To Latrea's advantage, she loved to read and began writing poetry and essays. She even won a number of essay contests. Writing not only served as an emotional outlet but also helped her self-esteem. Although she was two steps behind her classmates for the first few years of school, she caught up quickly. School was challenging only in the social sense; academically, Latrea was a star.

Middle school was harder on Latrea than elementary school because the main goal in middle school is to fit in, she says. You don't want to stand out. "When I was in middle school, it was hard because I was already different, whether I liked it or not. There was nothing I could do or say about it. My mom used to say that I tried to turn myself inside out to try to fit in," she says.

A girl who sat in front of Latrea in one of her high school English classes questioned her endlessly about why she looked the way she did. Several times, Latrea explained Pfeiffer's syndrome to the girl, but her explanation apparently wasn't satisfying. One day, the girl turned around and fixed her eyes on Latrea. "I don't mean any harm," she stated in a sassy voice, "but if I had a child that looked like you, I'd throw her away."

The words hit Latrea like a sucker punch — a sharp right that put her down on her back. Desperately, she tried to regain her senses, tried to get her eyes to focus, in case another insult was about to be launched her way. *If only the classroom floor would open and swallow me*, she thought. *Help me disappear.* Instead, she sat perfectly still, eyes straight ahead. Later, she would wonder whether, after a thousand seconds, she'd even breathed.

High school wasn't better. In 11th grade, one of Latrea's classmates picked on her every single day, and every day after school Latrea told her mother what the boy had done that day to hurt her. The taunting went on for weeks. At first, Donna told her to turn the other cheek. That didn't help. Then she told Latrea to tell her teacher, which she did, but the teasing didn't stop. Latrea went through the entire chain of command with no resolution. "No one listened," she says.

"I said to my husband, 'It ain't fair! I'm so tired of this! She has the right to go to school in peace,'" says Donna. She spoke to the teacher herself, but the taunting continued. At wit's end and against her husband's judgment, she finally told Latrea that if that boy picked on her again, she should knock him out. "I said, 'Then call me, and I'll come and get you,'" says Donna.

The next day, the boy and his friends started on Latrea again. Just as her mother had instructed, she balled up her fist and let him have it.

"I didn't realize that child would actually do that," says Donna. "My husband said, 'I told you,' and I said, 'I'm not sorry!'"

In the principal's office, the vice principal told Latrea that he'd have to call her mother. "I wouldn't do that," she said.

"Well, we have to call her," he replied, picking up the telephone and dialing the number. After explaining the situation to Donna, the vice principal finished by saying, "We're suspending her."

Donna's voice boomed over the phone's receiver: "Oh, no, you're not!"

Latrea smiled to herself. She not only stayed in school, but the boy also never bothered her again.

WHEN LATREA WAS ALMOST 20, she underwent her last surgery, a cosmetic procedure to try to build up her forehead. "I thought in my mind, if they could do all this other stuff, they could make me look normal," she says.

The day of surgery, Latrea was wheeled into the operating room at 7:30 in the morning. The procedure took much longer than expected and she lost a lot of blood. Rather than going to the recovery room afterward, she was taken straight to the intensive care unit. "The doctors were scared," she says. "It was kind of touch-and-go."

Afterward, she remembers her mother telling her, "Latrea, no more. The doctors said they've done all they can do; the rest has to come from you. You're never going to look like the average Joe walking down the street. That's the cold, hard fact. No matter how many surgeries you have, you're never going to look like anyone else. Find whatever it is inside yourself and pull it out of you. I can't watch you go through this."

During her freshman year of college, and for the first time in her life, Latrea experienced self-acceptance. "I finally realized, this is who I am," she says. She had been trying so hard all her life to be the same as everyone else. She had tried to fit in, to look like the other girls, to have a friend. Forget popularity. Forget being on the cheerleading squad. Never mind homecoming court. But to have a friend, to be liked for being the person she was. She realized that she'd spent the past decade consciously trying to be accepted by others. Trying harder wasn't going to change who she was. At that moment, she realized that if anyone was going to accept her, it needed to start with herself. She could move on from there.

I guess this is it, she thought. *I guess I have to take what I've got and work with it.*

Self-acceptance felt liberating to Latrea. "I didn't have to try anymore. I didn't have to put on a façade and be something I'm not. It's a lot harder to be something you're not. It takes so much energy," she says. When she realized that she was expending a lot of energy and not getting anything in return, it just seemed simpler not to waste the energy in the first place. "People just have to accept me for me," she says, "and if they can't do that, that's their problem."

She has considered having one more surgery to refine her forehead and straighten her eyes, but she's doubtful she'll go through with it. Her last surgery was traumatic, and there's only so much surgery can do. "Enough is enough. I've had everything under the sun and it didn't work. So I don't think anything will help. My eyes will forever be crooked," she says.

"People ask me, if I were to live my life over again, would I change anything? I wouldn't," she says. "I have no regrets. I've learned from my experiences. The experiences shaped who I am. I don't think I'd be able to appreciate life and the struggle of life without those experiences. People get caught up in the little things. Not many people say struggle is an opportunity, but with struggles, you gain something about life and something about yourself. I'm not against bettering yourself, but, at the end of the day, you still have to take what you have and make it work. Believe it or not, Latrea is not a bad person to be at all. I don't think I want to be anyone else."

EIGHT MONTHS INTO HER pregnancy, Latrea's blood pressure is sky-high. Her body, which is terribly swollen, isn't handling the pregnancy well. The doctor tells Latrea and her husband, Barry, that he might have to deliver the baby early. If Latrea has preeclampsia, also called toxemia, she and the baby may be in grave danger. He sends them immediately to the emergency room. It's two days before Christmas. In light of the baby's pending arrival, Barry is feeling particularly anxious. He has a stable job as an Equal Employment Opportunity assistant for the U.S.

Department of Defense but nevertheless worries that he won't be able to support Latrea and the baby. He wonders whether their disabilities will make a difference to his child. Barry has cerebral palsy, and he wonders whether he'll even be able to hold his baby.

LATREA MET BARRY WYCHE while she was living on campus at Gallaudet University in Washington, D.C., and working toward her bachelor's degree in psychology. After some online and telephone conversations, they arranged to meet in person.

Latrea took a train to meet Barry, but when she arrived at her destination, something didn't seem right. *Wait a minute*, she thought. *Did he say Springfield or Silver Spring?* Then her cell phone rang. "I'm here and you're not," said Barry. "I just wanted to touch base, to make sure you weren't going to stand me up."

She had boarded the wrong train. Springfield is in Virginia, and Silver Spring is in Maryland. She was in the wrong state.

"Don't leave!" said Latrea, as she scrambled to board the right train.

And he didn't. Not then and not later. Within about a year, they found themselves sitting together on the couch, talking about their disabilities and what they meant to their future. "I was naming all the things that could possibly go wrong with me," says Latrea. She told Barry there was a chance she'd be completely deaf, a chance she could be completely blind, a chance that he would end up having to take care of her. She asked him forthrightly, "Do you really want to get involved with me? Because if not, I understand."

Barry said he didn't care. She says, "He said he loved me for what I am. 'If it happens,' he said, 'we'll deal with it.'"

Latrea graduated from college in 2005, a year after Ashley started her first year of college. That fall, Barry and Latrea were married. When Barry read the vows he wrote to his bride, the whole congregation cried. "I think even the pastor was trying to hold back tears!" says Latrea.

BLOOD TESTS TAKEN TO find out whether Latrea had preeclampsia come back negative. Good news. Still, her body is finished carrying this baby, so her obstetrician schedules a C-section for December 27. Latrea and Barry are sent home to have Christmas with their families. Early in the morning of the 27th, they return to the hospital, and Latrea is prepped for surgery. Because her body is so swollen, the nurses can't find the spot to administer the epidural. They take turns, growing more frustrated by the minute.

"Bend over and crouch like a cat," one nurse barks.

"Do you not see what's in front of me?" says Latrea, referring to her gigantic belly. "I can't bend over and crouch like a cat!"

"Do you want us to help you or not?"

Half an hour passes. Finally a nurse hits the target. Now they must wait for Latrea to be sufficiently numb before beginning the surgery. While they're waiting, Latrea's doctor tells her that the surgery should only feel like pulling and tugging. She shouldn't feel any pain. The moment he begins the surgery, Latrea shrieks, "That doesn't feel like pulling and tugging! That feels like pain to me!"

Her doctor is unfazed. A few minutes pass. "How are you doing?" he asks Latrea.

"My intestines and guts are out on the table, but otherwise I'm okay," she says.

After more pulling and tugging, Latrea yells, "Is she out yet?" Not yet.

Latrea lashes out at Barry. "You did this to me! I'm lying here because of you!"

The nurse begs to differ. "You did this together," she says.

"Oh yeah? Well then, how come he's not lying here with me, with his intestines all over the table!"

Then, at 9:09 A.M., Olivia Danielle Wyche makes her entrance into the world. She weighs 5 pounds, 13 ounces, and measures 19 inches long. She's beautiful.

Olivia. Her name is Latin for olive branch, a symbol of peace. The moment Olivia is born, Latrea forgives Barry for his "transgression." Within a week, Barry will be holding the baby as though he was born knowing how, just as his mother-in-law told him he would.

"Every day is a journey," Donna told Barry, after he expressed his fear of being a father. "You walk through each one."

CHAPTER 9

not just another pretty face

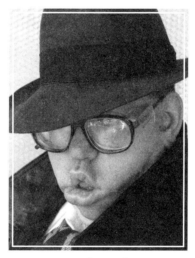

Matthew Joffe

When a man is singing and cannot lift his voice
and another comes and sings with him,
another who can lift his voice,
the first will be able to lift his voice, too.
That is the secret of the bond between spirits.

—Martin Buber, "Ten Rungs"

SOMETIMES IT'S JUST EASIER to trudge through the streets of Manhattan than to try to hail a cab, even on the darkest days of winter. One time, 13 taxicabs in a row stopped to pick up Matthew, but they took one look at him and sped away. Several times, he already had a grip on the door handle when the driver hit the accelerator. The sudden lurch of the vehicles stung his hand and stung his sensibilities. So he often walks, making his way up the center of the street, ignoring the honking horns and using his cane to help keep himself steady.

Because the street is better lighted than the sidewalks — street lamps are designed, after all, to assist drivers, not pedestrians — he feels safer walking there. He doesn't have night or peripheral vision, so the headlights from oncoming traffic help to light his way. During the winter months, he bundles up in his down overcoat, topped off by his Russian-style fur hat. From behind, negotiating the busy streets of New York City, he looks like Truman Capote. From the front, he is Matthew Joffe.

When Matthew was born in 1953, his mouth was wide open. His jaw hung down to his chest, says his mother, Florence. He stayed in the hospital for a few weeks, but he was sent home without much explanation or advice.

Because Matthew's mouth didn't close, he couldn't suck well enough to eat. He became very thin, says Florence, so she used her maternal instincts: She put her thumb on his cheek to stimulate chewing and somehow managed to get food into him. "It was touch-and-go for a while," she says. And, although they didn't get any answers from physicians, she knew one thing: "If he was going to make it, I could not treat him like a handicapped person."

When he was about a year and a half, Matthew exhibited other problems. He still wasn't walking and he had difficulty holding up his head. Sitting in his high chair, his head would slump forward or to the side. His left eye looked slightly off-center, and his right eye pulled to the right like a car in need of a wheel alignment. When Matthew did try to walk, his movements were awkward; he'd pick himself up only to fall down again.

His parents took him to a series of doctors, but they were told again and again that medicine did not have any answers. "Put him in an institution, because he'll be dead within a year," one doctor told them.

Eventually, a physician team at Columbia Presbyterian in New York City ordered a test for myasthenia gravis, a condition primarily characterized by progressive muscle weakness and fatigue (Aristotle Onassis would later die from it). When medication to treat the condition didn't help, the team ordered a "proof-positive" test, the results of which came back negative. By process of elimination, the doctors diagnosed Moebius syndrome.

A rare congenital nerve disorder, Moebius syndrome affects the sixth and seventh cranial nerves, although other nerves can be affected as well, causing a kind of facial paralysis. Because people with Moebius are unable to move their facial muscles, they can't visibly express their emotions. They cannot communicate surprise, fear, anger, happiness, disbelief, or dozens of other emotions just by facial movement. Emotions do not register on their faces. Their main communication panel — the face — is out of order.

Communicating with someone who has Moebius is like communicating via e-mail before emoticons were developed. Without the benefit of facial expression and tone of voice, messages can be ambiguous. For instance, if someone says "good" with a smile, the message sounds positive. If "good" is said with a frown and a strong tone of voice, the person likely means, "Well, it's about time!" If someone says "good" in a higher-than-normal pitch and with eyebrows raised, the message might mean, "Who cares!" Said with a wink and a certain tone of voice, the word is loaded with sarcasm. Facial expression is crucial to communication.

People with Moebius also have a certain "look" to them, as though their lips are puckered and open slightly. Often, they can't blink their eyes or close their mouth or lips completely, both of which also disrupt communication. Having open lips or an open mouth makes it difficult to speak clearly, especially with words using the letters *m*, *b*, and *p*, and may be interpreted as a sign of lower intelligence. In addition to communication problems, having an open mouth causes myriad health problems. An open mouth invites in bacteria, germs, dust, and pollutants that cause seasonal allergies, frequent colds, and a dry throat and mouth. An open mouth also encourages saliva to flow freely, which is embarrassing.

Matthew's parents were determined to get him as much help as possible. At age four, he underwent weekly procedures to stimulate his mouth electrically so that it might close. Each week, Matthew and his parents would make the long journey to the medical center, where the physician would place what looked like a microphone against Matthew's cheeks, sending an electrical current through his face. After many treatments, the physician hung up the device and told Matthew's parents that nothing else could be done.

Several years later, Matthew underwent a temporal fascia sling procedure, whereby surgeons took fascia (connective tissue) from his leg, threaded it through his skin below his jaw like a sling, and attached both ends to the sides of his face. The procedure was designed to bring his jaw up and away from his chest, not to solve the problem of his open mouth. Even so, his parents weren't giving up.

MATTHEW RACES ACROSS an open field. His pursuers are fast on his heels. *OWWWooo! OWWWooo!* Their primal cries cut through the air. His heart pounds in his chest, in his head, in his eyes. The flat landscape is empty. No trees, no hills, nothing but miles of land. *OWWWooo! OWWWooo!* My God, there's nowhere to hide! Arrows rip past him. They spear the earth. *Thwack! Thwack!* Up ahead, shelter! Matthew runs harder. He might make it! Sweat drips into his eyes, blurs his vision. "God, let me make it!" An arrow screams behind him. *Thwack!* He falls to the ground, still panting. The arrow opens his back like ripe fruit. Juice spills out onto the earth. *Gotcha!* The air is silent, and the silvery-white sky turns metallic gray. Miles away, a late summer storm looms. A spent arrow sticks out of the earth like a grave marker, and Matthew's racing heart slows until it beats no more.

It's a recurring nightmare.

AT ONE OF THE NEIGHBORHOOD baseball games, someone tapped Matthew on the cheek. At that moment, something happened that had never happened before: Matthew's mouth closed — and stayed closed for about 30 seconds. Then it opened again.

"It was the spookiest, most exciting thing that ever happened," says Matthew, who was an adolescent at the time. For the next several months, he, his parents, and various physicians tried to re-create that occurrence. At first, it was thought that the reaction was caused by an overabundance of calcium in his body (calcium affects how muscles work), but a blood test showed that wasn't the case.

The incident led to an experimental procedure to reestablish the muscle–nerve connection that, it was hoped, might allow his mouth to close. An incision was made behind his right ear and the skin was peeled back to expose the nerves and muscles. The area was wired with electrodes and systematically stimulated. "No one knew what to expect," he says.

The procedure worked to the extent that his nerves were stimulated, but there was trouble making the connection between the muscles and the nerves. There was some talk about implanting a type of pacemaker, but a connection couldn't be made between the nerves and the muscles that controlled Matthew's mouth. Matthew and his parents were told once again that nothing more could be done.

Something had caused Matthew's mouth to close for a half-minute; his parents reasoned that some kind of a connection between his nerves and muscles must exist. It was just a matter of finding it and somehow stimulating it to perform correctly. Even if the connection was like the proverbial needle in the haystack, what was the harm in looking a little longer, trying a little harder? His mouth had worked, if only for 30 seconds. That must mean that the capability existed for his mouth to function properly. It couldn't have been an aberration. Science wouldn't let them down.

Matthew's parents were tight-lipped in the car during the ride home. Their disappointment with the electrode experiment settled in their gut, every now and again rose into their throat, and was sharp to the taste. Matthew rode in the backseat, mouth open and eyes clouded with disillusionment.

That night and for many nights after, he would dream that wild Indians were hunting him.

BECAUSE OF THEIR INABILITY to move the muscles around their mouth, people with Moebius often have difficulty speaking. Matthew was no exception. "I sounded like a dishwasher going through the cycles," he says. "It was very harsh on the ears."

"When Matthew was diagnosed years ago, there was an assumption that the facial muscles were paralyzed," says Sara Rosenfeld-Johnson, a speech and language pathologist and founder of Innovative Therapists International in Arizona. Paralysis means that the signals the brain is sending to the muscles aren't being received and, consequently, the muscles cannot move. In that case, she says, "There's no reason to do any muscle exercises, because nothing will help."

Rosenfeld-Johnson discovered, however, that roughly 85 percent of people with Moebius syndrome have paresis, not paralysis. Paresis means the muscle cannot perform the action that the brain is asking it to do. The sensory signals from the brain are being received, but the muscles are either too weak or are simply untrained to perform their function.

"On the surface, they look the same because the muscle isn't moving," Rosenfeld-Johnson says. So how does one tell the difference? Rosenfeld-Johnson explains that a neurologist can provide a definitive diagnosis, but a simple screening test offers a pretty good clue. If your hand, for example, were paralyzed, you wouldn't feel someone touching it with a vibrator, but if a vibrator was placed against a muscle with paresis, you'd feel the sensation.

Rosenfeld-Johnson, who looks at how muscles function, created a unique style of oral-motor speech therapy she calls muscle-based therapy. She's careful to point out that this type of therapy doesn't replace traditional speech therapy; it is performed in conjunction with it.

For speech to be intelligible, a person must have the strength and endurance for normal muscle movement. People with muscle-based disorders often have poorly developed, weak oral muscles. Using an assortment of horns, straws, and bubbles (which the kids love "playing" with) in a hierarchy of difficulty based on resistance and exercise physiology, Rosenfeld-Johnson's muscle-based therapy works to strengthen and train these muscles. The therapy also serves to teach individual muscles, such as those that control the tongue and the jaw, to work independently. The first step is to strengthen the muscles enough so that patients can close their lips. Improving speech is secondary. (To make an "m" sound, for example, you first have to be able to close your lips.)

More than a decade ago, a young boy with Moebius was referred to Rosenfeld-Johnson. Because she knew little about the syndrome, she did some research. She found limited material, so when the boy walked into her office, she wasn't sure that she could help him. Nevertheless, she began working with him using her muscle-based therapy techniques and, to everyone's delight, he made tremendous progress.

Soon after, she was contacted by a woman from an organization hosting an international convention on Moebius in Canada. Rosenfeld-Johnson recalls, "She asked me to be a speaker, and I said, 'Whoa! I've only seen one child with Moebius!' And she said, 'You're the only one who's making any changes.'" So Rosenfeld-Johnson and her husband packed their bags and drove to Canada.

At the conference, she was struck by the facial similarities of the attendees. She also was struck by their love of laughter and witty use of language. "Because they don't have expressions to use, they have developed, across the board, an incredible sense of humor," she says, the same way a deaf person relies more heavily on vision or someone who is blind has intensified hearing. "They can't use facial expressions, so they use language."

Rosenfeld-Johnson spent the entire weekend getting to know the other attendees and evaluating children individually. By the end of the weekend, as she was saying good-bye to everyone and leaving the hotel, she caught a glimpse of herself in a mirror and was confronted with a non-Moebius face. "I was startled! My own face shocked me!" she says.

That first conference hooked her. She says, "I fell in love with them and their families that weekend." Today, she says, they're like family.

Rosenfeld-Johnson evaluated Matthew several years ago. If he were younger, ideally a child, she might have been able to help him. Her intuition and her experience, she says, tell her that the earlier a person with Moebius gets therapy, the better the results. She notes, "I'm working with a woman now who is 23, and the changes are minuscule and very slow."

When she can help people with Moebius early enough, the results are tremendous. Most of her patients experience total lip closure, retracted tongues, and normal speech. They are also able to eat more easily, without choking, and they don't have to use the compensatory patterns that Matthew uses for speaking and eating, although he's certainly successful. Also, because they can close their lips, they're more accepted by their peers.

Rosenfeld-Johnson trains other therapists to use her muscle-based therapy, not only for people with Moebius, but also for people with cerebral palsy, Down syndrome, Parkinson's disease, autism, and Fragile X syndrome — anybody with muscle-based articulation problems. She also serves as the international spokesperson for the Moebius Syndrome Foundation in the areas of speech and feeding and is beginning to expand her international work.

She offers some advice if you find yourself in a conversation with someone you're having difficulty understanding, particularly if the person has facial paralysis: Don't look at the mouth. The visual information you get when you look at the speaker's mouth is confusing, she says, and makes speech harder to understand.

Few people would have difficulty understanding Matthew speak. Letters that require teeth on the lips (f is an example) or require the lips to meet (such as m, b, and p) sound guttural, but they're certainly recognizable. For ten years, Matthew had specialized speech therapy, where he learned a sophisticated tongue-tip placement system that allows him to speak the way he does today. He brings his voice up and away from the bottom of his throat and catapults it forward, using his tongue to form words the way most people use their lips.

Having a voice gives people the ability to dispel notions that others have of them based on their appearance. For example, someone with cerebral palsy may look so physically disabled that an onlooker may assume he or she is mentally challenged as well. Because of the lack of facial expression, people with Moebius syndrome sometimes are considered mentally disabled. If people who are in a wheelchair or are hearing-impaired are able to have a social exchange or conversation, expressing their opinions using verbal skills or some other form of understandable communication such as sign language, they have the ability to engage other people. Suddenly, someone who might have been overlooked can make a connection. Having a voice, verbal or otherwise, helps establish us as thinking and feeling people.

"Speech therapy gave me my voice, literally and figuratively," Matthew says. "That's a powerful gift." By having a voice, he could meet the world head-on.

In junior high, Matthew and his loyal friend, Steven, ate lunch together every day and sometimes hung out after school. One day, three guys ganged up on Steven in the hallway, taunting him because he ate lunch with Matthew. Steven was a chubby kid who spent most of his time reading schoolbooks. He certainly was no thug, but when the fists began to fly, he returned fire. When all the boys were sent to the principal's office, Steven faced suspension.

Matthew heard what had happened and marched down to the

principal's office. "I'm here about Steven," he said. "I don't condone fighting, but it's not fair to punish Steven because he defended his decision to have lunch with me and be my friend." The principal was stunned and thanked Matthew for his loyalty. "We won't suspend him," he said.

That incident validated for Matthew that the voice he had from years of speech therapy was a gift indeed. "I spoke out on my behalf. I was a survivor." But it meant even more than that: "I'd make it in life."

Not only did Matthew master speaking English, but he also majored in French and psychology in college. One of his psychology professors had a tremendous impact on him, acting as a mentor and unofficial private tutor during Matthew's junior and senior years.

"I was invited to his home for dinner. We would argue words in his office that would best represent the translation from French to English. It was an education you do not get in a classroom," Matthew says.

MATTHEW'S RIGHT EYELID doesn't close; it's even difficult to blink. Called ptosis, the condition causes numerous eye problems. Our eyelids and eyelashes serve crucial functions, including protecting our eyes from dust, bacteria, and sunlight; keeping them moist; and allowing them to rest. The ability to blink and keep the eye moistened is vital to the health of the cornea, which can become ulcerated without this ability and result in vision loss.

People with ptosis often experience irritated eyes and eye infections. When Matthew was nine, surgeons tried to fix his right eyelid. But, like the experimental procedure to get his mouth to close, the surgery was unsuccessful. Three years later, he reluctantly underwent a double eye surgery at Columbia Presbyterian Hospital to reposition both his eyes toward the center of his face. His fear of losing his vision was almost overwhelming. Matthew made his surgeon promise not to cover both his eyes after the operation; he needed to be able to see out of at least one eye.

Children who undergo multiple surgeries usually have an accelerated childhood. In other words, they grow up quickly and have a keen sense of their own mortality. Whether it's the first surgery or the 17th, there isn't much difference in the anxiety level. The routine may be familiar — the pre-op tests, the needles and IVs, the reassuring gestures of hospital staff and family members — but the notion of being anesthetized and perhaps not waking up afterward is terrifying every time.

PEOPLE WITH MOEBIUS SYNDROME sometimes have anomalies of their hands and feet, such as clubfoot or webbed fingers. Matthew was born with a clubbed left wrist, for which he sought treatment as an adult. During an office visit, Matthew was waiting in the exam room for the doctor. Several of the doctor's residents came in to observe.

"There were three or four of them," says Matthew. "They were like paparazzi; they all came in at one time and were jockeying around me to get a good angle."

Matthew's doctor silently entered the exam room and noticed the residents staring at Matthew's face. "People!" he announced loudly. "Remember, we're here about his hand."

With clinical — and curious — eyes, the residents were examining the posture of Matthew's mouth, the angle of his eyes. Did they ask his permission? Did they wonder how their staring might make Matthew feel? Did they think they had carte blanche because they were doctors? Matthew and many people with disabilities spend more than their share of time wondering how others perceive them. They wonder what people are thinking. Are they afraid? Will they reject me? Rarely does someone ask about their feelings. Rarely if ever does someone say, "Am I making you uncomfortable?"

Matthew was relieved when his doctor entered the exam room and broke up the crowd, even though he expects that type of response from people. He admits, matter-of-factly, "I'm not just another pretty face."

WHILE ONE DAY BROWSING in a poster store in New York City, Matthew saw a ghost. Situated among a group of prints, an abstract in green and gray gave him a shiver. "The print is right out of my nightmares," he says, "the place where all my battles were fought. If I could jump inside the picture, I'd be that little kid running for cover and not being able to escape. It's autobiographical."

The landscape that offered nowhere for Matthew to hide now hangs in his apartment, standing out enough from the rest of the artwork — Dutch Masters, etchings, and whirling dervish art — that guests comment about it, although he never offers an explanation. The print simply serves as a reminder of his fears.

"Once I realized that those fears would always be with me, the grip they had on me loosened," he says. "Like opening a door. I think I knew that by buying it, I could achieve mastery over the nightmare. I could get in it and I could get out of it. It's not my future, it's not my present. It's my past."

"I HAVE TO TELL YOU something," said one of Matthew's friends during college. "From the first time I met you, it took a long time to look at you and be comfortable."

His friend's confession spurred an epiphany for Matthew. "I was thinking, not 'You son of a bitch,' but 'That took a lot of courage and nerve.'" Matthew realized that if he could bring his appearance to the fore right away, maybe he could be accepted more easily. He also echoes the sentiment of others whose differences, facial or otherwise, prove stumbling blocks. "Once he got to know me," he says, referring to his friend, "he stopped looking at me the same way."

It's true. Once you know someone, you stop *looking* and begin to actually *see*.

"There's such emphasis on surface beauty — the fashion industry, media, Hollywood. Looks are everything. People with our conditions fail miserably at meeting the standards," says Matthew. "People don't realize that just because we look different doesn't mean we don't want the same things."

Are not love, acceptance, friendship, and even a smile some of the easiest things one human can give to another? "We're all alike," Matthew says. "Just the packaging is different."

Trained as a psychotherapist and educational therapist, Matthew is director of the Office for Student Services at LaGuardia Community College, City University of New York. Among other things, he counsels students and designs programs, in-services, workshops, and training. As a frequent public speaker, Matthew takes a cue from his college friend and opens his presentations by talking about his appearance. "I know you think I look funny," he'll say. "Guess what? I look funny! Let's agree and move on."

He and his audiences are at ease because the cards are on the table. There's no need to pretend that he's not different or to shy away from him. By announcing his difference, he controls the dynamic. He introduces himself to his audience on his own terms.

As a learning disability specialist, Matthew counsels young adults in academic, career, and personal matters. He helps people discover and reach their potential. He thrives on the immediate feedback he gets from students and the quick results of his work. Each graduation ceremony is proof of his efforts.

He remembers one young woman who wasn't doing well in her studies. She couldn't pass her biology class, and she came to Matthew, crying. He counseled her and helped her discover a field of study for which she was better suited. Years later, she called Matthew to tell him she'd continued her education and was teaching special-education children in Brooklyn. Over the telephone, he could tell, "she was smiling from ear to ear." If not for him, she said, she wouldn't have made it.

MATTHEW LEANED AGAINST the front of Baccarat, one of his favorite shops in the city. It was Memorial Day and he was lost in thought, waiting to catch the bus that would take him to see friends for dinner. Two kids, probably about 12, ambled past him, snickering to each other. Matthew thought, *What else is new? You don't think I know what you're snickering about? You don't think it's happened a hundred times — several hundred times — before?*

The boys stopped about 25 feet from Matthew. Suddenly glass exploded at his feet. He quickly covered his face. The empty bottle the kids hurled at him smashed into the stone base of the building and shattered. A glass arrow. Matthew looked up and saw two wild Indians running toward Park Avenue.

Matthew leaned hard into the building. *The streets are unpredictable. You never know what can happen. You never know what someone might do to you,* he thought. The world quieted as he carefully assessed whether or not he was okay. Then he gripped his cane, swept the glass away from his feet, and boarded the bus.

MOEBIUS SYNDROME IS extremely rare. "No one knows the exact incidence of Moebius," says Vicki McCarrell, who co-founded the Moebius Syndrome Foundation in 1994. "We do know that in the U.S., we have about 900 with Moebius on our mailing list, another 100 from Canada, and a few thousand in support groups around the world."

Throughout nearly his entire adult life, Matthew had never met anyone else with the syndrome. For 40 years, he was alone. Then he learned about an organization through New York University called Forward Face that he considered joining. "He told me about it and I encouraged him to do it," says Florence, who had insisted Matthew go away to college when he was 18.

"That was the hardest thing I ever had to do," she says. But she did it purposely. "I wanted him to be on his own." She recalls dropping Matthew off at college; she and Matthew's sister were in tears. As they were driving away, Mr. Joffe checked the rearview mirror, then turned to his wife and said, "I don't know what you are crying about. Look at him!" Both she and her daughter turned around and saw Matthew standing in a crowd of young men, shaking hands and talking.

The Forward Face office is just about ten blocks from Matthew's apartment. Through Forward Face, Matthew met a young woman who also had Moebius, who in turn introduced him to the organization's support group called Inner Faces. At the urging of the young woman, Matthew agreed to attend an Inner Faces meeting. It was January 1994 and the snow was flying. When he arrived at the meeting, he discovered it was a planning session for the group's first stage production, something he hadn't quite bargained for.

"I thought, 'I have to figure out how to get out of here!'" says Matthew. Then a woman walked up to him and congratulated him on his courage. "You're so courageous to come here and not walk away," she said. How could he walk out after that?

Jodie Morrow, the group's advisor, remembers Matthew walking through the door, wearing his Cossack hat and snow-dusted overcoat. "He made quite an impression," she says. Later that evening, as Matthew was leaving, he told Jodie, "Today was a watershed day," and she remembers thinking, "Who is this man?"

That was the beginning of his experience with Inner Faces. Jodie and the production team were planning a theatrical piece, called *Let's Face the Music*, designed to drive social change. They promised that the members wouldn't feel embarrassed. Their goal was empowerment, not ridicule. "That meant a lot," says Matthew.

Just weeks before opening night, Jodie called Matthew and told him he was going to sing the male vocal lead for the theme song. The man who had been slated to perform was ill. Matthew said, "You're crazy!" But Jodie doesn't easily take no for an answer. On opening night, Matthew went on stage alone and walked off a changed person, discovering that deep down, he is "a camera hog."

"He loved it more than anything," says Jodie. "It was a very special thing for him."

As part of the piece, the Inner Faces group performed a "mirrorlogue," which is a monologue performed in front of an invisible mirror separating the performers from the audience. In the mirrorlogue, the performers talk to the mirror, honestly and openly addressing the feelings they have when confronted by their own reflection.

During rehearsal, Matthew wasn't sure whether he could pull it off. "I was scared," he says. "My heart was racing." He enjoyed writing the mirrorlogue, but because his face doesn't move, he didn't think he could convince an audience that there was a mirror between him and them. "I couldn't relate to a mirror," he says. "It was beyond my comprehension."

When it came his turn, one of the production's consultants looked at him and gave him a handheld mirror. "Here, talk to this," she said. In that instant, he felt completely understood. Matthew would later write about the experience: "Identity requires finding the right mirror to see yourself correctly." Through Inner Faces, he found that mirror.

Later that evening, he and a friend walked to the East Village to get dinner. Out of the late October evening mist, a tide of devils, whores, thugs, and monsters arose: the Halloween parade. Years before, Matthew had been brutally ridiculed by a group of people in their Halloween garb, Indians in full headdress. Since then, he had loathed Halloween, but this day was different. "Oh, it's Halloween," he said, realizing it held no meaning for him. Its power was lost inside that mirror he'd held up like a magic wand.

Let's Face the Music, which was performed off-Broadway, has a scene called Masquerade, for which the players created masks of their faces. The goal was to lead the audience into the experience of discrimination, prejudice, and oppression, says Heather Gary, an artist who led the mask-making workshop. Everyone in the audience would feel the harshness and intensity of the players' experiences. No one would leave the performance unaffected.

Heather instructed the players how to study what happens to the anatomy of a face when people feel rage, sorrow, grief, or fear — emotions they relate to oppression — by looking at photographs of faces, studying the anatomy of a face, and playing with different facial expressions in a mirror. Finally, using gauze, plaster of Paris, and paint, each member would create a mask that expressed a strong, unique experience of oppression. The exercise filled Matthew with dread.

Everyone else in the group was playing with different expressions in the mirror and crafting masks. He couldn't do it. He knew what the anguish inside him felt like, but he didn't know how his anguish should look on his mask. He was unable to make the leap, he says, from a face that's expressionless to a mask full of expression. "I was stuck in my own body," he says.

"In his heart, he so wanted to explore it," says Heather. "It was really beautiful that he had strength and confidence to ask me for help." So Heather worked with him to create a mask and, in the end, he did make a powerful mask, one that was truly expressive. "He hung in there. It took a lot of guts," she says.

On stage, the players danced with their masks on until a thunderous voice blunted their mood. The voice taunted them, pointed a finger at them. The players froze into postures of strife, grief, or fear, or they cowered on the ground, afraid. There was nowhere to hide. Suddenly, Matthew was gasping for air, running across an open landscape, a band of wild Indians in hot pursuit. "That's where I had my meltdown," he says. The jeering voice made him wince and he shut his eyes tight. "It was really raw."

Then the music slowed, became gentler. The players turned in their masks of anguish and held up plain white masks to their faces — masks that signified a rebirth from oppression, an undeveloped self taking its first breath after being born again. The masks were expressionless, symbolizing the purity and potential of the human spirit, and the sense that we're all the same. "When you come out of oppression, it takes a while to form and know who you are," says Heather. "There's a lack of sense of self, an undeveloped person who needs to be developed."

Finally, they removed those masks and introduced themselves to each other, as if for the first time. Behind the mask is a person. The mask is only the way we recognize each other. Sometimes, our masks don't at all reflect how we imagine ourselves to be. Sometimes, our masks belie our true selves.

Heather, who is one of the founders of Inner Faces, believes mask-making helps people explore a variety of issues on a universal human level. Sometimes the fun that comes from mask-making opens conversations or helps open a window of understanding. Mask-making and other forms of art therapy help people discover their value and, Heather says, answer the question "How do I create a meaningful life when society wants to judge me and write me off?"

WHEN MATTHEW WALKED IN on the first Inner Faces meeting, he immediately tried to think of a reason to leave. Not only did he stay, but through the years, he has also served as the treasurer, vice president, and president of the organization, which is more like a family, a community. "It's a wonderful place to go to be yourself," he says. "No one expects an explanation of why you look a certain way. They simply welcome you."

The group uses the video it produced to educate others and build acceptance. They've shown the video to high school health classes and encouraged dialogue with the students. Because he's good at it, Matthew opens the presentations, challenging the students to ask questions from their "hearts and minds" and to not be afraid to get to know them.

During one presentation, Matthew noticed a young woman in the audience who sat like a stone throughout the entire video. She was motionless, barely breathing. She showed up in another class to watch the video again, sitting down next to Matthew in the audience. Before the video started, Matthew shared some of his experiences of being facially different, the challenges of getting people to see past his exterior, to give him a chance, to not be cruel. The young woman listened intently and then, without warning, exploded into tears. She felt awful, she said, for even thinking that a pimple on her forehead was significant. In the time it took to show a video and hold a discussion, one person was changed. Remembering that moment, Matthew says, "It was a pure, unadorned connection to another's person's soul."

Matthew had experienced something similar years earlier. "In college, all my friends would come to me to discuss their relationships," the questions ranging from mild to graphic. "I was baffled because I was no relationship expert! They'd ask me about sex," says Matthew, a robust laugh spilling out of his otherwise quiet face. "I'd say, 'You're the one doing it; I'm just reading about it!'" Finally, one of his friends confessed, "I'm coming to you because you won't judge me."

MATTHEW STRUGGLES WITH several physical limitations. "Not that I was ever an Olympic contender, mind you," he says. The muscles throughout his body are weak and his balance is compromised, which is why he walks with a cane. He is unable to raise either of his arms above his shoulders or hold them stretched out at his sides. Carrying anything of substantial weight is out of the question, so he often relies on friends or delivery services to bring him groceries and other necessities. He wishes he could be handy around his apartment, but lifting a hammer or stepping on a ladder to reach something is too difficult. His physical limitations make him feel vulnerable.

He says, "In our society, we have a caste system of disabilities. Some are more accepted than others. I've had friends in wheelchairs or who needed crutches, and people are able to look at them and draw a quick conclusion: 'Oh, he was in a car accident, or he had polio.' But when they look at someone with a craniofacial condition, they're confused. It's hard for people to get past it. It's almost like the face becomes disembodied from the rest of the self and that's all someone sees."

Matthew's journey to accept himself has led him to question his masculinity in the face of his disability and limitations. "Do I see myself as a disabled individual? Does my disability prevent me from being macho? I can't hammer a nail. I don't drive. I don't do 'guy things.' I don't have notches on my belt to represent people I've slept with."

With the help of a therapist, Matthew was able to understand that disability doesn't preclude masculinity. By taking an inventory of the things he does that are valuable, he was able to redefine masculinity and apply it to himself. He learned that his life isn't defined by whether he gets married or has an intimate relationship with a woman.

Instead, he says, "It was about living my life on my terms, doing what I want to do, and forging a life that's satisfying without those things. I don't know if it will ever happen. The longer I go without, the harder it will be to have. For me, the biggest problem is taking a risk with a woman."

When Matthew was four, the little boy who lived down the street ran away from him. Matthew ran home crying. His parents told him it wasn't about him but about the other boy. His mother told him, "Understand one thing about life: People staring is not your problem, it's theirs. You have enough of your own problems."

That helped him not feel responsible for what happened, but it didn't help soothe his sorrow or his anger at being rejected. Years later, that boy would tell Matthew that he'd been afraid of catching his "disease." Rejection paralyzes the heart, even a heart that so deeply wants to love and to be loved.

People have told him how lucky he is not to date because love can be so painful. "It used to infuriate me," he says. "I want to be in the experience. Why should I be left out? I want to have a good time in my life and make it the best I can. I'd like to meet someone wise and mature and open enough to consider me in a relationship. I want to know what it's like for someone to embrace me and not run away. That's really what I want."

Through Inner Faces, Matthew met a woman named Caroline who was several years younger and worked as a nurse. They would go to the theater, museums, restaurants, and movies together. Matthew loved her sense of humor and her gentleness, the way she always thought about others before herself. They were regular companions and when they weren't together, they'd spend hours talking on the phone.

Caroline was one of the founding members of Inner Faces. She had neurofibromatosis, a rare disease characterized by tumors in the connective tissue, skin, and bone. By the time she met Matthew, her disease had progressed to her lung. She was on chemotherapy to treat it.

One of Matthew's best memories is going to her house with another friend and spending hours just talking and laughing. "A couple days later, she had a seizure," says Matthew. He knew right away what that meant. The cancer had attacked her brain. Chemotherapy was no use because it couldn't bypass the blood–brain barrier, the brain's natural defense against "foreign" invaders. Her prognosis was not good. "She knew that I knew," says Matthew, and that was enough. They never talked about it.

As Caroline got weaker, she had to be hospitalized. Then late one evening, Caroline's mother called Matthew. "Come to the hospital if you want to say good-bye," she said.

Caroline was in a coma by the time Matthew arrived. She looked so peaceful and innocent. He pictured her smile, struggled to hear the sound of her laughter. Standing at the side of her bed, Matthew took her hand and kissed her forehead. "Go in peace," he said. A few hours later, Caroline died.

After the funeral, Caroline's sister-in-law hugged Matthew and whispered in his ear, "You know that she loved you."

When Matthew was a young boy, every nightly newscast on New York's ABC affiliate station ended with the same song, played to an image of the 59th Street Bridge, brilliantly lighted against a backdrop of Manhattan. The music haunted him, amplified his losses, reminded him of his loneliness. Later, when he felt sad, the song's melody would play in his head. One day the song played on the radio. For the first time in his life, Matthew heard the title: the "Forget Me Not Song."

All of us, from time to time, reflect on the past. What could have been, had we done things differently? Made certain decisions earlier, later, or not at all? Not been afraid? Matthew wishes he and Caroline could have had more time together; wishes they had taken better advantage of the time they did share; wishes they had dared to disturb the universe.

"I still miss her," he says.

ALTHOUGH HE DIDN'T FIT into any groups as a child or young adult, Matthew has been involved in both Inner Faces and the Moebius Syndrome Foundation since 1994. He's currently vice president of the Moebius Syndrome Foundation's board of directors.

"It's a kind of fuel for the spirit, seeing how I can make a contribution and seeing what I can get back," he says. "Being involved with the Moebius Foundation and Forward Face keeps me going, keeps me alive. In a way, it has softened some of the pain of being alone. As much as I like being by myself, it's hard to be alone."

Inner Faces participated in a photography project a couple of years ago with former high-profile New York fashion photographer Rick Guidotti. The shoot was part of Guidotti's not-for-profit project called Positive Exposure, which seeks to challenge people's notions of physical difference and beauty and offer people with differences a positive, uplifting experience. Since 1998, Guidotti has been photographing people with various genetic conditions, though his primary focus is albinism.

"I'm using albinism as the metaphor because it's instantly identifiable as being different and there's a cultural reaction to the condition, sometimes positive but usually negative," says Guidotti, whose early work was featured in *Life* magazine.

"I was always forced to work within the parameters of the beauty standard. It used to drive me crazy as a visual artist," he says. Then one day, he saw a young girl with albinism boarding a bus and he thought, *She's beautiful!* Realizing she'd never been included in the traditional beauty standard, he got the idea to redefine beauty. He travels the globe, challenging the stigma of difference with his photography. He makes presentations to health professionals and children in elementary and middle schools to celebrate the spirit of diversity.

Guidotti tells of a teenage girl with albinism who came to his studio for a shoot. "She walked in, shoulders hunched, head down. This kid had zero, absolutely zero self-esteem," he says. "She was tortured and teased her entire life. And she was beautiful!"

He turned on his fans, cranked up the music, and went into fashion photography mode. "The studio exploded!" he says. "Her head went up, her hand went on her hip, she was bouncing all over the place! Right in front of the camera, she became empowered. And no matter what would happen in the future, she had the weapon of self-esteem. And it is sustainable," he says, adding that the experience helps people to move from self-acceptance to self-esteem to self-advocacy.

Another young girl confided to Guidotti after a shoot that she was changed by the experience. She said she realized the hatred and abuse she experienced every day would never disappear, but what had disappeared was the hatred she felt for herself.

Before the Inner Faces shoot, Matthew and a friend were in Matthew's apartment, standing in front of his open closet, talking about what he should wear. Matthew remembered looking at the men's fashion supplement in the Sunday *New York Times* years earlier and thinking, "I can't wear this stuff." Instead of being able to put himself in the magazine photographs, Matthew saw only his disability. But his father, who was in the textile industry, taught him how to buy clothes and over the years, Matthew changed his perception about dress. Eventually, he felt comfortable buying fashionable clothing for himself because he had reached a point where he saw himself in a different way. That was about to happen again.

He and his friend sifted through his clothing. What colors would look best? Would formal attire be more appropriate? Should he choose stripes or stick with solids? Suddenly, Matthew burst out laughing and said to his friend, "Do you realize that we're like a bunch of women?"

When Matthew arrived at the studio, he began to feel nervous about the shoot. In the past, when he looked at photographs of himself, he had wished his face showed the emotions he was feeling. He overheard Guidotti talking to the others while he was shooting them, saying things like "Show me feeling. Show me happiness. Show me sexy." How could Matthew express himself? He couldn't show those things, at least not through his face, and he told Guidotti so.

Guidotti was unfazed. "I said to him, 'You have more attitude in your little finger than anyone I've ever photographed!' He was concerned he didn't have the expression, but everything he does is full of expression. Matthew is extraordinary. He's the greatest guy on the planet."

So Matthew took the risk and said, "Photograph me as though I were a *New York Times* fashion model." And that's just what Guidotti did. By tilting Matthew's hat this way and that, turning up his collar, and encouraging him to express himself through his posture, Matthew's personality — his playfulness, wit, and joie de vivre — emerged. Wearing a leather bomber jacket and brown fedora, Matthew was a fashion model. A female member of Inner Faces, wearing a chic red dress and holding a long-stemmed rose between her teeth, joined Matthew for a tango while the camera clicked away.

Through the photography project, the members of Inner Faces not only got to live out a fantasy, but they also learned about themselves, to see themselves a little differently. The goal, says Guidotti, is for every person to look into a mirror and say, "I am amazing!"

"It was a riot!" says Matthew, adding that the group is trying to raise funds to host a gallery exhibit of the photographs. "Sometimes, it takes someone else to get you to see something in yourself," he says and, after a moment of reflection, "I did look good, if I don't say so myself!"

※

CHAPTER 10

finding kim

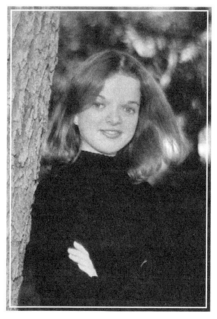

Kim Nuss

O brother man! Fold to thy heart thy brother.

—John Greenleaf Whittier, hymn

"W HAT'S WRONG WITH YOUR daughter's face?" the young woman asked Pat as she watched her five-year-old daughter splash around in the kiddie pool. On that steamy July day, Pat Nuss was happy to cool off at the community pool with her two children, Kim and Jon. Pat didn't blink. "Oh, she was born with a genetic defect called Crouzon's. She's already had two major surgeries. She had her first surgery when she was six months old." Pat went on to explain that craniofacial reconstruction had to be done in stages. It was a matter of time and patience, she said.

Most mothers wouldn't have reacted so kindly to that blunt question. But Pat, who taught high school math and science at the time, says she was in teacher mode and just wanted people to understand her daughter's condition. "It didn't bother me and I didn't hesitate to explain," she says, adding that by sharing information you reassure people, particularly young mothers who might be afraid, rightly or wrongly, that their child could "catch" something.

The Nusses had just moved back to Nebraska and had settled in a small community of fewer than 5,000 people. Since they were the newcomers, people wanted to know who they were and because Kim had a craniofacial condition, the family stood out even more. "People are curious," says Pat. But until that time, Kim had no idea she looked different from everyone else.

PAT WAS 36 WHEN she became pregnant with Kim. Because of her advanced age, she underwent an amniocentesis to check for chromosomal abnormalities, especially Down syndrome. The test results showed nothing abnormal. When Kim was born, Pat says, her obstetrician suspected something was different about the baby, but he couldn't pinpoint it. Kim's forehead was flat and her eyes appeared to be set far apart. Pat and her husband, Jerry, thought that Kim's head might be a little misshapen. "Her head looked funny," says Jerry.

Pat's obstetrician referred the family to a geneticist from Omaha.

When Kim was six weeks old, the geneticist examined her but couldn't offer a definitive diagnosis. "Come back when she's six months old and we'll do skull X-rays," he told the family. "In the meantime, monitor her development." So for the next several months, Pat and Jerry watched Kim carefully and observed that she was developing normally, like any other healthy, ordinary baby, even if she still didn't look quite "right."

"She looked different, but I didn't think she looked that different. When they couldn't really give me a definitive diagnosis, I thought, well, there must not be anything horribly wrong. I guess I was in denial," recalls Pat.

In August of that year, when Kim was just about six months old, she caught pneumonia and was hospitalized. While she was in the hospital, her pediatrician took skull X-rays and sent them to the geneticist. They determined that the spaces between the bones of her skull, called sutures, were closing prematurely. Kim had craniosynostosis.

The bones in a newborn's skull are loose to provide flexibility when the baby moves through the birth canal and to allow for brain and facial growth after birth. When the sutures close too early, the skull expands in the wrong places and can appear quite deformed. Surgery to open the sutures was needed right away; otherwise, Kim's growing brain might not have anywhere to go, and the function of her eyes and ears also might be affected.

At the same time, the geneticist gave the family a definitive diagnosis: Crouzon's syndrome. Crouzon's syndrome is genetic, although spontaneous cases do occur. The syndrome is chiefly characterized by craniosynostosis and abnormal fusion of the facial bones, which results in wide-set, bulging eyes (sometimes to the extent that children cannot close their eyes completely), a small nose, and a flattened mid-face. Some children with Crouzon's experience hearing and vision loss as well as problems with the cervical (upper) spine. Like children with Pfeiffer's syndrome, which is a cousin to Crouzon's, the underdeveloped mid-face section often leads to breathing difficulties and problems with jaw alignment, which typically can be addressed as they grow. The lower jaw grows at a normal pace, seemingly unaffected by the syndrome. But the upper jaw, or maxilla, is part of the mid-face and is stunted, resulting in an outward-jutting lower jaw.

Like Pfeiffer's syndrome, Crouzon's has an autosomal dominant inheritance pattern; thus, an adult with Crouzon's has a 50 percent chance of passing on the syndrome to a child. The syndrome is caused by a genetic mutation in the fibroblast growth factor receptors (FGFRs) on chromosomes 4 (FGFR3) and 10 (FGFR2). FGFRs are responsible for connective tissue, skin, and bone growth. Because the genes that cause Crouzon's have been identified, genetic testing for the syndrome is available.

Kim was admitted to Children's Hospital in Omaha for surgery. The neurosurgeon explained how she was going to cut into Kim's tiny skull and reshape the bones. After the surgery, Jerry was shocked at the sight of his daughter's face. Her eyes, the size of golf balls, floated on top of her bloated face. "I was scared as hell," he says.

JERRY WAS TRANSFERRED when Kim was a year old and the family moved to Denver, Colorado. Within a year, Kim would need to undergo a second surgery, a procedure to reshape her forehead and give it better curvature. The surgery would involve making an incision along the coronal suture that runs along the top of the skull and connects the frontal (forehead) bone with the two parietal bones that together form the top and sides of the skull. The incision would extend across the skull to the tops of her ears and above her eyebrows. The frontal bone would be removed, reshaped, and reattached. The surgery would be complex. Jerry and Pat were focused on the risks; with the surgeon cutting into their daughter's skull, so close to her brain, many things could go wrong.

Several days before the surgery, Pat's anxiety was at an all-time high. She showed up at the surgeon's office unexpectedly one day. He took her into his office and showed her before-and-after photographs of some similar surgeries to help put her mind at ease. "One that stood out was a boy whose eyes were almost on the sides of his face," says Pat. "He showed me the before picture and the after picture, and I thought, 'Oh my gosh, this guy's good. He's really, really good.'"

To everyone's relief, Kim's second surgery went smoothly, but while she was recovering in the pediatric intensive care unit, a little boy in the next bed had a severe reaction to anesthesia and went into cardiac arrest. The medical staff worked frantically to revive him, but their attempts were futile. He had been in the hospital for a tonsillectomy — an ordinary, run-of-the-mill procedure. Although the boy's reaction to the anesthesia was extremely rare, the scene was humbling. Recalls Pat, "You take for granted that everything is going to be fine."

WHEN KIM WAS FIVE years old, her family moved to Aurora, Nebraska, a town about 25 miles east of where Kim spent the first year of her life. By this time, the symptoms of Crouzon's were beginning to show on Kim's face. The midsection of her face had fused and stopped growing in proportion to her forehead and chin. Her eyes bulged, and her nose looked as if it had sunk into her head. Now away from the children and families she'd been around for several years, who were accustomed to her appearance, she found herself a strange being in a strange land. Everyone stared at her. Children pointed at her. The kids at school taunted her. "Why are your eyes so wide? Why don't you have a nose?" She was called hammerhead and flatface. The teasing was relentless. "Yeah, you! You with the stupid face! Why do you look that way? You're ugly! Why does your nose look that way? You look like someone punched you. What's wrong with your eyes? Your smile is crooked. You're ugly! I can't stand to look at you! You make me sick!" Most nights, Kim wet the bed. Many mornings, she didn't feel well enough to go to kindergarten. Moving, her parents told her, was out of the question.

Kim was a smart girl, though, and she somehow got the idea that if she were active and social, she'd be part of some groups and naturally make friends. From kindergarten through high school, she joined groups and clubs, and participated in sports. Softball became a passion, starting with the first time she whacked a plastic Wiffle ball off a tee when she was six. As a teen, she played on a summer softball team, and she played to win. She joined Girl Scouts and 4H. She went camping and fishing and took piano and dance lessons. She made friends. "Thank goodness she was very independent and very confident in her abilities," says Pat.

Still, Kim was unhappy with how she looked. "I tried to ignore it, because it made me really unhappy to look at how I was different," she says. "You know you look different and that's all you really think about. You try not to. You do typical girl stuff: comb your hair and put your hair in pigtail braids. I wore the typical fashions of my age. I just tried to do the best I could with what I had."

Kim's craniofacial doctor was still in Denver and every two years, the family made the 800-mile round-trip for a follow-up appointment. When Kim was nine, the school nurse told the Nusses about a new craniofacial clinic at Children's Hospital in Omaha, which was less than 130 miles from their home. A new surgeon, Dr. Richard Bruneteau, was establishing a craniofacial team. The Nusses made an appointment.

When Dr. Bruneteau walked into the exam room, he immediately introduced himself to Kim, shook her hand, and said, "I want to learn more about you."

"He totally ignored Mom and Dad," says Pat, with a laugh.

Dr. Bruneteau, a gentle man with a wide smile, said to Kim, "I understand you have Crouzon's syndrome. Tell me about it." She did, and then he said, "I would like you to be my patient if you would consider me as your doctor."

Afterward, Pat and Jerry asked Kim what she thought. "He treated me like a real person," she told them. "I thought it was really cool that he talked to me. I'm the one who's going to have to have the surgery, not you guys." Dr. Bruneteau later told Kim's parents, "I could just tell she's the type of person who wants to know what's going on."

He recommended performing what's called a LeFort III mid-face advancement on Kim. The procedure is designed to bring the entire mid-face forward by separating the bones in the face from the skull, then moving them forward into proper position. "It makes more room for the eyes in their sockets, realigns the teeth, and makes the central face more prominent," says Dr. Bruneteau. Although the procedure itself has been around for several decades, the techniques to perform it have been modified over the years. "It's an operation that continues to evolve," he says, adding that it's not performed everywhere.

During the meeting, Jerry said, "This must be a dumb question, but have you done this before?"

Dr. Bruneteau replied, "I've done these things with people's noses. I've done these things with their eyes. I've done these things with their foreheads. I've done these things with their mouths. But I'll be honest, I've never done them all at the same time to the same person."

The Nusses liked Dr. Bruneteau and Kim felt comfortable with him. It was worth a shot.

THE PROCEDURE COULDN'T BE performed on Kim for a few years in order for her to finish receiving orthodontia work. In the meantime, her facial development was monitored through skull X-rays and CT scans, and Dr. Bruneteau's craniofacial team began planning the procedure.

The surgical team, which included Dr. Bruneteau, neurosurgeon Leslie Hellbusch, and oral/maxillofacial surgeon Michael McDermott, did the planning well in advance. "You have to look at a lot of different things," explains Dr. Bruneteau. "You have to look at how the teeth are going to fit together. You have to have a psychologist involved, because you're going to be changing the way someone looks. Obviously, you have to have a geneticist involved on the front end and sometimes a speech therapist, although Kim didn't need one. A lot of different disciplines are needed to take care of a child with a craniofacial problem. The surgery itself is difficult because of the nature of what you're doing. You're moving someone's face."

The team met as a group, reviewed X-rays, and mapped out the operation, even going so far as practicing the procedure on a model.

Eighteen months of preparation went into Kim's surgery; they wanted to be sure that each member of the team knew who was going to do what and when. "We literally choreographed the operation," says Dr. Bruneteau. "If you don't, you have a long operation that turns into a longer operation."

SURGERY WAS SCHEDULED FOR the end of June 1994, when Kim was 12 years old. She had been waiting for that day for years, the magical day when she would be transformed — when she would get the face she was meant to have, not the one she was born with. What would she look like after surgery? She would look perfect, she thought, and no one could ever tease her again.

Before the surgery, Kim kept very busy. She spent the first part of the summer at camp and as soon as camp was over, it was time for her surgery. There was no spare time to think about it or let it keep her up at night, she says, though in the back of her head she kept thinking about how perfect she would look afterward. At her preoperative visit, Kim was fighting a cold and a slight fever, so the procedure was put off for another month, until July 21. After 18 months of planning, Dr. Bruneteau wasn't taking any chances.

"I was disappointed because all the preparation was in place," says Kim. Getting ready for this major surgery involved not only technical details, such as arranging for overnight accommodations, but also mental preparation. Besides, a month seemed a long way off. When you're 12 years old, time is an inchworm with nowhere to go.

On the day of Kim's second preoperative physical, Pat remembers Dr. Bruneteau sitting down with them to explain the risks. "Kim, I want you to know up front what risks there are," he said. "What's the worst-case scenario? You could die. Or, because we're opening up your skull, you could be brain damaged; because we're working with your eye and optic nerve, you could be blinded; because we're using bone grafts, you could get an infection and we'd have to start all over. I want you to be aware of all these things."

"In the meantime," says Pat, "my husband and I are sitting there with tears in our eyes because he's painting a pretty clear picture."

Dr. Bruneteau continued. "You know I'll do everything and anything. I have a great team of doctors, and they wouldn't be on my team if they weren't the best. But I want it to be your decision, not a decision your mom or dad or I can make. If you don't want to go through with it, that's fine. If you're scared, that's fine. But I do want you to be aware of the risks."

"I remember not wanting to hear that," says Kim, who quickly came up with several reasons she shouldn't worry about the risks. "If I died, I figured I'd be dead, so it wouldn't matter because I'd be dead. I wouldn't even know I was dead. Or I figured, how could I look worse? Why would we be seeing this doctor if he wasn't any good? Of course he's going to do a good job. That's his job. If I worried about it, it wouldn't mean it would be less likely to happen." Her decision was to stay the course. For years leading up to the surgery, Kim had told her parents, "I don't always want to explain why I look different." She knew what she wanted.

Kim looked Dr. Bruneteau squarely in the eye and said, "I've been waiting years for this. Let's go for it."

Her parents weren't so sure. Jerry, who ordinarily keeps a cool exterior, was visibly shaken. If it had been his decision, he says, he's not sure what he would have done, but he knew Kim wanted the surgery. "I'm glad I didn't have to make that choice," he says. Pat closed her eyes and saw the little boy in the Denver hospital, on life support after his tonsillectomy. "Everything is going to be fine," she kept telling herself.

During the weeks leading up to the surgery, Pat was feeling more and more tentative. She asked herself endless questions: What are we doing? Are the risks worth it? Did it make sense to trade a risk of brain damage for the chance to have Kim's face blend in better with most of humanity? She wondered whether it was okay to let Kim make such an important decision. On one hand, it was her life, her face. Kim was eager to be the person she felt she was meant to be. The surgery was important to her. On the other hand, she was only 12 years old! She couldn't fully understand the magnitude of the risks. What if the knife slipped and Kim suffered brain damage? What if the surgeon cut too close to the optic nerve and she lost her vision? She would be in surgery for at least ten hours. What if her body couldn't handle that much anesthesia? What if she had to be placed on life support? What decision would Pat and Jerry make? The what-ifs multiplied exponentially inside her until one day she choked on them. At that point, Pat knew she had to let go.

"There's the saying, 'Let go, let God,' and I did," says Pat. "I talked to our minister and said this is what we're facing and he said, 'We'll be with you every step of the way.'" Her faith in God and the promise of prayer from friends and family were an immediate relief to Pat. "It's one of those things where you get strength from a higher power." Even if you don't have a strong faith, she says, you just have to let go.

"The day of surgery, I had a million things to do," says Pat. "I took music, quilting, crosswords." Jerry, who relaxes by walking outdoors, spent a good part of the day outside the hospital, pacing back and forth.

IN THE OPERATING ROOM, the show was about to go on. This day was the culmination of months and months of planning and rehearsing. Everyone knew their lines, their steps. Lights, props — everything was in place. Dr. Bruneteau started by making an incision across the top of Kim's head, along the coronal suture (the same place the incision was made for the surgery to reshape her forehead when she was two). He lifted the skin from her forehead and pulled it over her eyes to allow Dr. Hellbusch, the neurosurgeon, access to her skull. He needed to take a piece of bone from Kim's skull to use elsewhere.

Separating bone from the skull is dangerous, says Dr. Bruneteau. Surgeons performing this type of work essentially are using carpentry tools and are working two millimeters — 0.08 of an inch — away from the brain. One slip of a tool can cause uncontrolled bleeding, brain damage, or, worse, death. Dr. Hellbusch removed a slice of bone from the top of Kim's skull and split it. Drs. Bruneteau and McDermott made an incision along the lower eyelid to expose the lower portion of the orbit, as well as the cheekbone region.

Next, Drs. Bruneteau and McDermott separated Kim's eyes from the bone, 360 degrees, all the way to the optic nerve. "The face is only attached by the optic nerve and the tissue that's posterior to it," says Dr. Bruneteau. In other words, once the tissue around the eyes was cut, the eyes were tethered only to the optic nerve. The risk of injuring the nerve by stretching it or causing severe swelling in it was very real, and the result might be that Kim would lose her vision. Once the eyes were separated from the bone, the surgeons made a series of cuts throughout Kim's mid-face to separate the bones, as well as an incision inside her mouth to separate the soft tissue from its underlying bone. The goal was to move the center of Kim's face forward, and they would accomplish this by first separating the upper face from the lower face. Next they would separate the right half of the face from the left half at the base and bridge of the nose.

With Kim's face pulled apart in this manner, the risk of infection was tremendous. These spaces, explains Dr. Bruneteau, typically are sterile. They ordinarily aren't open and exposed to bacteria. But in the case of surgery, bacteria easily can be introduced, resulting in terrible infections such as a brain abscess, meningitis, or a bone graft infection. To reduce this risk, time in the operating room is kept to a minimum and lots of antibiotics are given to the patient, both before and after surgery. Still, Dr. Bruneteau and his team wouldn't know until some-time during recovery — or even much later — if Kim were to get a seri-ous infection.

Once the bones were separated from each other and the soft tis-sue was disconnected from the bones, Kim's facial bones were pulled forward nearly an inch into a normal position. Dr. Bruneteau grafted some of the bone harvested from Kim's skull to her cheekbones to build them up, as well as to patch the hole in the skull from where the bone had originally been taken. He used the rest of the harvested bone, along with a variety of metal plates and titanium screws, to reattach the pieces of Kim's face in its new position. Finally, the incisions were closed.

Eleven and a half hours after the surgery was over, Drs. Bruneteau, Hellbusch, and McDermott came out to tell Pat and Jerry that their daughter was fine. "I was sure relieved, I'll tell you that," says Jerry.

Then Dr. McDermott said, "Thank all your family and friends for their prayers." Pat looked up at him, puzzled. He continued, "I can always tell when God is with us."

Pat says, "I just cried."

The next step was recovery. Remembering that young boy in the Denver hospital, Pat knew that Kim wasn't out of the woods yet. Kim was moved to a bed in the pediatric intensive care unit, right next to a young girl who'd been in a car accident. One of the girl's family members brought her a stuffed Simba, from *The Lion King*. When Simba's paw was squeezed, he'd say, "I'm trying to be brave like you!" The Nusses had seen *The Lion King* with close friends just a week before and were admiring the toy, so the next day, the girl's family brought Kim a stuffed Simba. Kim loved the toy, but its message meant more to Pat. "I was trying to be brave, like she was," she says.

Just a day after surgery, Kim was eager to see herself. She wanted to touch her new face. It was nighttime when she finally had the energy to make her way out of bed. The lights in her room were turned down, but the hallway lights beamed a path to the bathroom. Inside, there was no need to turn on the light; she could see well enough. "I knew that I wouldn't be 100 percent perfect right away," she says. She looked into the mirror. Her right eye was swollen closed; rows of sutures, thick with dried blood, looked like tiny caterpillars clinging to her face; and her long hair, save a section in the back that could be pulled through the back of a baseball cap, was gone.

Oh my God, she thought, *it's so beautiful!*

Kim's jaw was wired shut and would stay that way for nine weeks following the surgery. Because she couldn't speak, her parents felt it was important that one of them be with her at all times while she was in the hospital. Pat stayed during the daytime, and Jerry spent the nights in the reclining chair next to Kim's bed. She was never left alone. If she needed anything, she'd clap her hands to get her mother's or father's attention. Jerry knew that Kim was feeling better after just a couple of nights when she clapped her hands and then handed him a handwritten note that read, "Did you know you were asleep?"

Kim was released from the hospital on a sizzling July day. Unlike most people who have been in the hospital for more than a few days, she wasn't all that eager to leave. She says, "I was really apprehensive about going home. I didn't feel good at all and I was scared as hell to leave the hospital. I liked my hospital bed. I liked having the doctors and nurses there in case something happened. You're safe in the hospital."

At the front entrance to the hospital, Kim climbed out of her wheelchair and into the backseat of her parents' van. Inside was an oppressive heaviness, and Kim, with sweat already dripping down her forehead, struggled to catch her breath. The ride home took about two hours. She wasn't feeling confident. Every muscle in her body ached, her scalp felt as though it was on fire, and when she squinted to keep the sun out of her eyes, her eyebrows screamed. Every bump in the road sent shock waves through Kim's body. She felt like a squirrel stuck on an electric fence. *One more hour till we're home*, she told herself at one point. Through her wired jaw, she whimpered and moaned. All of a sudden, the back of her throat filled with saliva, and her stomach began to heave. *I can't throw up!* she thought. *I can't open my mouth!*

Pat heard Kim gagging in the backseat and yelled to Jerry to pull over. Luckily, they were just approaching a rest stop, so he turned off there. Kim's mouth was full of vomit, and there was nowhere for it to go but down her throat and back up again. Pat rushed Kim, who was crying, gagging, and coughing, to the rest area bathroom, where she eventually flushed the vomit out with water. Nobody had warned them that this might happen or what to do if it did. "The doctors can't predict everything," says Kim. After that incident, Kim wondered what else might happen. How she regretted leaving the hospital!

Once home, Kim worried about her tracheotomy. When she took out the tube, she had an open wound the size of a quarter, a gaping hole that led directly to her lungs. "What if I drop a quarter in there? I mean, I knew I wouldn't, but what if I did? How would I get it out? It freaked me out," she says.

She slept sitting up in a chair for the first week because of all the draining and swelling in her head. She learned to like puréed food (noodles and tangy spaghetti sauce taste great, she says, and also Eggo waffles with peanut butter and a little milk). She learned to favor button-down shirts rather than pullovers. "You never know how hard it's going to be," she says. "They teach you the big things, but it's the little things that bring you to your knees." Things like trying to pull a shirt over your head and feeling as though your scalp is being ripped apart. Finally, after about a week, Kim was glad to be home and eager to settle into the life of a regular teenager.

KIM'S PARENTS WERE THRILLED with her recovery and the results of the surgery. "I could tell the difference the minute she was wheeled out of the operating room," says Pat. "You could see the cheekbones. You could tell right away. It just made such a difference."

"I thought she really looked nice," says Jerry. "I think it was better because she felt good. We're thankful that she had it and that everything turned out all right."

Since Kim's surgery, a newer technique called distraction osteogenesis has been developed. The procedure helps avoid one portion of the traditional surgery. Dr. Bruneteau explains that all the bony cuts are performed, but the surgeon doesn't pull the face forward and reattach it with plates and screws. Rather, after the surgery, the patient is fitted with external headgear that slowly stretches and pulls the face forward. One of the main benefits is that distraction osteogenesis can be performed at a younger age; there's no need to wait until the child is an adolescent and done growing. Another major benefit is a reduced risk of infection, because bone grafts aren't required.

Although Kim's surgery was a success, it wasn't 100 percent perfect. Kim's right eye, which was swollen shut after her surgery, never reopened. Eventually, Dr. Bruneteau removed a slice of her eyelid so that her eye would open and she could see; the flip side is that her eye doesn't close all the way. Because her eye wasn't used for so long, it became lazy, so Kim now wears eyeglasses. She also had her nose reshaped to remove a little crook in it. But to Kim's mind, these were minor blemishes. By this time, she'd already become accustomed to her face, and she loved how she looked. Her dream of looking normal, of never having to explain why she looked different, had come true.

While out one evening with some friends, an acquaintance approached Kim and said, "People keep asking me why your face is different. I tell them you had surgery." Kim's focus narrowed on the woman. *What! People are asking you why my face is different?* She couldn't understand why this person would say this to her. Because Kim was satisfied with how she looked, she sometimes forgot that she didn't look perfect. "I would be crazy to think no one would notice there was a slight difference in my face," she says. But the comment sent her sailing back to when she was a child, slamming her down into a schoolyard in Aurora, where the voices of children taunted her. She kept her eyes focused on the woman in front of her as she processed what a single person had said to her and then decided it wasn't worth thinking about any longer. "I really kind of had to let that go."

KIM WAS EAGER TO get on with her life after surgery, and for several years she avoided the topic altogether. She was tired of talking about the surgery, tired of being asked about it. Even talking about it more than once or twice a year was too much. All her life, she had just wanted to fit in, but for her first 12 years, she lived in shoes that were not fashionable. They fell far short, too far outside the norm. She was ridiculed and rejected. "I remember one time at the swimming pool and a lady walked up to my mom and said, 'What's wrong with your daughter's face?' It makes you uncomfortable and puts you on the defensive. It makes you feel like you shouldn't have to explain it every day for someone you meet for five seconds. Why do I need to explain it?" she asks.

Then one day, she slipped into shoes that looked a lot like everyone else's and suddenly people were kinder. No one asked probing questions. No one stared at her. Yet, on the inside, Kim knew she hadn't changed a bit. She was Kim because of who she was on the inside, not because of how far apart her eyes were set or the shape of her nose. Had she not been made to feel like a freak, the idea of undergoing surgery to change her appearance might never have entered her mind. Her difference would have been akin to having green eyes instead of blue or having blond hair instead of brown. But that's not how her life unfolded, and for years she was torn between an old self and a new self, trying to reconcile the two. Do you stuff your former self into an old shoe box and bury it in the backyard on a moonless night? "That whole concept is a freaky kind of thing to happen," she says.

Kim had been split between two worlds. She had run from one as fast as she could as soon as she could, but once she felt safe and took a moment to catch her breath, she turned around and started a tentative walk back again. "I'm getting more and more involved in that life, whereas all I wanted to do before was leave it. Baby-stepping backward helped me come to terms with it."

KIM GRADUATED FROM the University of Nebraska and is planning to be an art teacher. She's nearly comfortable with who she was then and who she is now. "I think it will take me a little longer to get 100 percent," she says. "I think I'm at about 90 percent."

Taking control of her experience and reliving it on her own terms have helped her gain ownership of it. For a college English class, she wrote a paper about Crouzon's, her surgery, and her experience. All the students were required to present their papers orally to the class. When Kim started presenting hers, she realized that each word of the story belonged to her. She directed the story line and the voice that told the story was her own. *I own this. This is mine*, she knew.

"I can explain it when I want now," she says. "My mom documented everything; she saved doctors' notes and photographs. I really appreciate it now. It allows me to talk about what I've been through on my own terms." If someone asks, she can pull out the scrapbook and the souvenirs from her journey — her stuffed Simba, hospital wristbands, get-well cards, all the notes she wrote when her jaw was wired shut, and the locks of hair saved from every single surgery — and say, "Here you go. See you in an hour."

Being in control of her own story, as well as being comfortable with the young girl she once was, has another important meaning. As Kim considers her future, she can't help seeing a small child who looks the way she once did. She has a 50/50 chance of passing on her condition to her children. She's given a lot of thought to those odds, wondering how important it is not to pass on the genetic mutation or whether it really matters what one looks like. But she thinks it does. "I would feel the burden of passing the gene on," she says.

From consulting with a geneticist on Dr. Bruneteau's team, she learned what her options may be. One is in vitro fertilization with pre-implantation genetic testing. After eggs have been harvested and fertilized with sperm, the embryos are tested for the mutation. Any with the mutation are destroyed and a healthy embryo is implanted in the uterus, with the option of freezing any remaining healthy embryos for the future. While there's a guarantee the baby wouldn't be born with Crouzon's, any number of other things might go wrong, of course.

"It's crazy to think about," she says. "You go through all that stuff with genetic testing and then your kid has something else." But that's true for all of us. Lightning strikes, sometimes twice. Kim also could choose to use a donor egg or to adopt a child. Another option, she says, is to just do it the old-fashioned way and take her chances. She was heartened to learn that if she did have a baby with Crouzon's, chances are the child would not have symptoms more severe than her own.

Her geneticist also told her that the world of genetics is moving pretty quickly and everything may be different five years from now.

Thinking about the future ensures that Kim won't forget her past. "You wish you could leave it completely in the dust, but at the same time, I appreciate the fact that it probably did make me stronger," she says. "People look at blessings as curses and curses as blessings, and you never really know what it is. I don't know if I'll ever really know. I can only imagine if I were drop-dead beautiful, I'd probably end up a snooty, snobby, stuck-up person, maybe thinking I was better than everyone else. I really think the whole experience grounded me and made me get to know myself better, too. I realized who I really was and what was important to me. I really think, too, that by looking different, it forced me to explore my other abilities. I had to rely on being able to talk to people, not being shy. I don't know if I would have been shy or not, but it forced me to try new things. What did I have to lose?"

In July 2005, Pat and Kim attended the North American Craniofacial Family Conference, sponsored by AboutFace USA and cleftAdvocate. At first, Kim wasn't interested in attending, thinking that to go to the conference would feel like taking a stampede of backward baby steps. But despite the high intensity of emotion involved in being there (Kim says she sobbed every single day), meeting the kids and the families made her realize that she has a great opportunity to share her experience.

When Kim was young, she never met anyone else with Crouzon's or with a similar facial difference. She didn't have the benefit of someone giving her practical advice, such as what might actually taste good when your jaw is wired shut for nine weeks that feel like nine months and how to make peace with the incessant whir of the blender. It felt good to be able to offer that kind of help and hope to others.

"I saw a ton of people with Crouzon's at the conference and I thought, wow, this would have been great to have when I was a kid. I met a girl who was having surgery soon and I said, 'You're going to look like me when you're done.' I'm glad it changed me like that. I can help people now."

Since coming home from the conference, Kim has toyed with the idea of using her artistic talent to portray people with facial differences, people not considered beautiful. "All artists paint normal kinds of people," she says. "You don't see huge noses or giant ears or no eyes. It would be very interesting to paint faces with Crouzon's or Apert's or tumors."

To stress asymmetry. To capture the texture of skin that's been touched by fire. To experiment with the way the light hits the contours of a jawline affected by disease. To disregard with abandon divine proportion, the mathematical ratio applied to facial features that helps define beauty, and to accentuate the humanity in all of us — imperfect and beautiful.

⁕

CHAPTER 11

our child, our heart

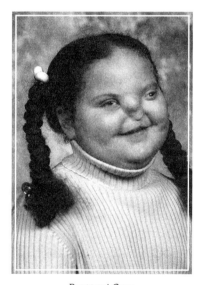

Bryttani Gore

I have loved the stars too fondly
to be fearful of the night.

—Sarah Williams

THE NEWS INITIALLY CAME as a shock, even though Casey Gore had been terribly worried all along that something was wrong with her unborn baby. Beyond normal anxiety or first-time-mom jitters, she had a gut feeling there was a problem. The women in her family had a history of high-risk pregnancies and miscarriages. Several babies had been born prematurely or with low birth weight, and some were stillborn.

When Casey was 24 weeks pregnant, she had her first ultrasound. Her doctor detected a cleft lip in the fetus and recommended she have a level 2, or three-dimensional, ultrasound to learn the extent of the birth defect. Two weeks later, Casey had the level 2 ultrasound, which showed that the baby had both a cleft lip and palate. Although the doctor who'd performed the tests wasn't sure how severe the defect was, she strongly urged Casey to consider terminating the pregnancy. She told Casey she was unable to tell whether the baby had a nose, and both of the eyes looked questionable. Later ultrasounds detected that all the baby's internal organs were on the opposite side from where they should have been. Still, Casey had no intention of terminating her pregnancy, so the doctor tried to prepare her for the worst, cautioning that there might be other things "going on" and that the baby she'd been carrying for just about six months might be born dead.

On September 29, 1998, four weeks before her due date, Casey delivered a 4-pound, 13-ounce baby girl at a hospital in Christiana, Delaware. The baby, given the name Bryttani, announced her birth by screaming at the top of her lungs. Despite this show of strength, the hospital staff didn't expect her to live long. She was born with a severe midline facial cleft that began at her lip and palate, extended through the area where the nasal structure should have been, and ended in the area of her left eye, which was missing. One of the physicians told Casey that if she were to shine a light through Bryttani's cleft palate, because of her absent nasal structure, she'd be able to see the fluid around her brain.

The cleft also involved her right eye (the gap in the structure of the eye is called a coloboma) and its optic nerve. She was born with a stub of tissue between her eyes and, as the earlier ultrasounds showed, mirror-image organs. This rare condition, called situs inversus, was the least of everyone's worries; surprisingly, it typically doesn't cause any problems. One of the doctors also said Bryttani was totally blind and deaf.

Bryttani was shuttled off to the neonatal intensive care unit and hooked up to an array of monitors. Only her parents, a black man of 23 and his 19-year-old white girlfriend, were hopeful.

The baby was born on a Tuesday. That Friday, the doctor finally allowed her to be fed through a nasogastric tube inserted into her mouth because of her absent nasal structure. "They said they didn't think she'd tolerate feeding," says Casey. "It was hard to see her not being fed." She tolerated the formula so well, though, that the next day the hospital staff tried a Haberman feeder, a bottle uniquely designed for babies with cleft lip and palate. Still, with just one airway — her mouth — Bryttani was at great risk of aspirating the formula and suffocating. Even her own saliva was a hazard.

As the medical staff went about their duties, Casey, wide-eyed and waiflike, sat in the nursery, rocking her daughter. She caressed her baby's cheek and smoothed her downy hair, looking beyond the tiny bulge on her forehead, the deep notch in her mouth, and one missing eye, and seeing instead a beautiful gift.

After ten days, the baby was discharged from the NICU. The doctor who discharged her said he was doing it against his will, but there wasn't anything more he could do for her. "They all thought she would not survive," says Casey. They released Bryttani so that she could go home to die.

CASEY HAD BEEN 13 when she moved out of her mother and stepfather's home and into her aunt and uncle's home, where she stayed until she graduated from high school. She got a job selling Kirby vacuums and met Marcel Gore. They became friends, often playing pool together, and started dating. Although their relationship wasn't serious, they discussed having a baby together, wondering what it would be like and thinking it might make sense to wait. But in January of 1998, Casey became pregnant. In a sense, Bryttani was planned, says Casey. She just arrived a little early.

Casey essentially was put out on the street after she became pregnant. She had no one close to talk to or to advise her. Marcel's family took her in, but they were new to her and there was no real relationship, no rapport yet. Casey comforted herself by thinking about her baby. *That's all I need*, she thought. *Even if nobody else in the world loves me, my baby is going to love me.* But then, after learning about all of Bryttani's health problems, she felt as though she was standing in a doorway, peering out at an empty universe.

"The hardest thing was not being able to pick up the phone and cry my eyes out to them," she says of her own family. Instead, she prayed.

Throughout Casey's pregnancy, her older sister kept their mother informed about the baby's health, but it wasn't until some months after Bryttani was born that Casey learned that her mother wanted to see the baby. So, after about a year apart, Casey and her mother, Debbie Lascola, saw each other again, and Debbie welcomed her daughter and granddaughter with hugs and kisses. "She told me that she missed me," says Casey.

The year of feeling alone and dealing with her baby's difficulties gave Casey strength. Now, when she's by herself in the hospital, waiting for Bryttani to come out of surgery, she's okay. "I don't need anybody to be sitting here with me because I know that the family loves her and that they pray over her. I look at it as that year gave me the strength that I have now. That's the past; it's done, it's over with. There are no grudges," she says.

Casey has the right attitude. The past is like an old man who follows you forever, more of a nuisance than a threat, really. It's only when you look back too often that you risk stumbling.

BRYTTANI WAS DISCHARGED from the NICU with home health care. A nurse visited the house twice a week to weigh the baby and check on her medical status. Through the nurse, Casey learned about a day program that would take Bryttani. Called prescribed pediatric extended care, the program is staffed by nurses and certified nurse assistants and is designed for medically fragile children. The children who attend PPEC have access to all types of therapies and an early childhood educator who helps them prepare for school. Each child is assigned a primary nurse who is responsible for the overall coordination of care.

Bryttani went to PPEC until she started full-day pre-kindergarten classes. Her primary nurse was a tremendous resource for the family, always making sure the baby had speech therapy and was gaining weight appropriately. "Anytime Bryttani had surgery, her nurse was on the phone, following up with the plastic surgeon and the team as to what care she would need. We were blessed because we had PPEC as our backbone," says Casey.

When Bryttani was three years old, she experienced a febrile seizure, convulsions brought on by a high fever. She was at the day program when she suddenly lost consciousness and began twitching violently. The staff called 9-1-1 and the paramedics rushed Bryttani to the emergency department. When the attending physician got a glimpse of Bryttani, he recognized her face immediately.

"She's alive," he said, just above his breath.

"Yes," said Bryttani's PPEC nurse, who was standing nearby and overheard him. "I've had her since she was seven weeks old."

"I discharged her from the NICU," the doctor said. "She wasn't supposed to live."

Casey laughs when she thinks about it now. "She's always proven everybody wrong," she says, to which Marcel adds, "They said she wouldn't see. She sees little things that I can't see! I think she surprises a lot of people."

Bryttani must have inherited that trait from her parents, who are now married. "A lot of people didn't expect us to stay together, even after I became pregnant with Bryttani," says Casey. "We've had our times, as everybody does, but I feel that it brought us closer together because it made us more focused. It calmed both of us down and we stick beside each other, and it's made us both stronger. We haven't done any of the stupid things that young parents do. We put Bryttani's needs first." Even when money is tight or when Casey and Marcel feel overwhelmed, they remember their pledge: Bryttani's needs come first.

Their determination and commitment to their daughter have kept them together, truly against all odds. "How well the family copes with the birth of a child who isn't healthy is directly related to how well each parent handles his or her own emotional response and supports the other," says Dr. Kathy Kapp-Simon, a nationally known pediatric psychologist with Northwestern University and the Cleft Lip and Palate Institute of Shriners Hospital for Children, Chicago. She has worked with children with facial differences for more than 25 years. Each parent may have to deal with a gamut of tough emotions, such as guilt, blame, depression, anger, and shame. Recognizing and appreciating those feelings are important steps toward moving beyond them. That Casey and Marcel were able to prepare emotionally for their daughter's medical problems before she was born was a blessing, they say, and probably contributed to their commitment to stay together.

Dr. Kapp-Simon recommends that parents also recognize what strengths each of them has and capitalize on them. That's just what Casey and Marcel have done. Casey has taken the lead in coordinating Bryttani's medical care, taking her to appointments with doctors, dentists, ocularists, and a low-vision specialist, most of whom are in Philadelphia, about a two-hour drive from their home.

"If it's a major appointment, like to talk about an upcoming surgery or something major, then he'll take off and come with us," Casey says of her husband. Marcel is a mechanic and part owner of a shop, giving him flexibility to take time off, and his parents have been at Casey's side for nearly every one of Bryttani's surgeries. For his part, Marcel gives Casey and Bryttani emotional support and encouragement, especially before a surgery, and pinch-hits for Casey when she's sick or just needs a hand.

THINGS COULD HAVE TURNED out much differently. Before Bryttani was born, Marcel wasn't working and, by his own admission, was more interested in doing his "own thing." But his daughter's impending birth changed him. He remembers thinking that he wasn't going to be like a lot of other people who "up and disappear," and says, "I wanted to make sure she was taken care of. She would have been taken care of if I would have had to work four jobs or five jobs."

Not all fathers of children with disabilities see it that way. Sometimes a man with a child who has an illness or disability that's not easily fixed may isolate himself and shut down emotionally. He'll keep his feelings to himself, often not even sharing them with his wife. He won't talk about his special-needs child to his male buddies, especially if they have normal children. He'll often shift his focus to work, where he can be successful.

It's a tough agenda to get over, says James May, retired director of the Fathers Network. Men have an image of what fatherhood should be and how kids should look; when their experience falls outside the norm, it becomes a struggle. "The truth is, men really do get isolated and they do get forgotten a lot. Men don't get a chance to talk about their experiences very often and probably don't have many avenues to talk about their losses and their grief," he says.

May says the limited research on how fathers deal with a child's disability shows that men take much more time than women to accept the reality of a situation. "They stay longer in denial," he says, "especially if the child is a son. They bring different dreams and issues to sons than daughters."

When May was running a Saturday morning network (really a classic support group, but called a network for the benefit of the men), a man called regularly, telling May that he was going to come to the group. The man called and called for two years, but he never attended.

May was puzzled by his behavior, but he knew from experience that persistence and patience are imperative. After all, May couldn't coerce the man into attending the group; he could only encourage him.

During one of the Saturday morning networks, May looked out the window and spotted a man sitting in his car. He wondered whether that was the man who'd been calling him. *I'm going out there to see if that's him*, he thought. Sure enough, it was.

"Why don't you come in?" May asked him.

"I'm really scared," the man confessed.

"Why?" asked May.

"I'm scared I might cry."

Although understanding a man's need to look strong, especially in front of a group of other men, May told him, "So far, no one's ever died from crying. Come on in."

It turned out that the man's daughter had profound cerebral palsy. He felt that if he joined the group, it would mean he would have to accept his daughter's disability. Intellectually, he understood that she had CP, but the thought of "going public" with it would cement her disability firmly and forever into reality. With encouragement, the man tentatively followed May inside. The other men were happy to welcome him and give him support. They encouraged him to tell his story, and no one even blinked when he sat with his head in his hands and cried.

"Once they get there," says May, "they're usually okay." Most of the men find the network a great experience, a place where they can be comfortable and accepted. "Sometimes, the humor gets wacky, irreverent," he says, laughing. "But that's how the men deal with it."

The Fathers Network was born from a graduate project by a couple of students at the University of Washington in Seattle in the early 1980s. The program caught on and grew, eventually moving to Bellevue, a suburb of Seattle, and becoming a program of the Kindering Center, a birth-to-three neurodevelopmental center serving children with special needs. Today, the Fathers Network offers resources and support to fathers and families who have children with special healthcare needs and developmental disabilities. The statewide program is funded by the Washington State Department of Health, foundations, and private donations. Similar programs for fathers are beginning to develop in other states.

One goal of the network is to help educate health-care providers and children's agency staffers so that they can do a better job of engaging fathers. "A lot of agencies aren't father-friendly," says May, adding that the essential belief is that mothers are the experts about their children. "They often hold IEPs [individual education plans] when fathers can't be there," such as on weekdays during the day, when the father is usually at work. In many families, with or without a child with a disability, economic factors dictate that one parent stay at work, usually the father, while the other takes off work for the appointment. By developing a family-friendly schedule, the network allows both parents to attend important meetings that involve their child. "Even at intake, if the social worker can make an attempt to have both parents there, it makes a huge difference," he says.

The next step is to actively engage both parents during meetings and appointments. May has found that even when the fathers are in attendance, many staffers don't direct questions to the father or even make eye contact with him, leaving him feeling unimportant and unneeded. When May trained staff about their expectations for fathers and their involvement, they often told him that they had never even thought about it.

Encouraging fathers to be involved with their children is especially important now, because many more are eager to be in that role. In the last several years, May has noticed a surge in fathers desiring full involvement in their children's lives. They are no longer satisfied with being the breadwinner and provider; they want to help support their children emotionally, from being present and vocal during medical appointments to talking openly with them about their feelings.

Of course, this isn't true for all men. Some shut down completely and some run away. May says, "There's no question some men won't get over it. But I'd like to think that early on, if someone contacted them and told them they were important to the child and to the family, they'd be there."

CASEY AND MARCEL BELIEVE things happen for a reason: "We feel that we were given a very special child with very special needs." They've made a point of always telling Bryttani that she is special. Because of her positive attitude and outgoing nature, she does well in social settings. "She doesn't really give people a chance to stare at her," says Casey. "As soon as she makes eye contact with someone, she says, 'Hello, my name is Bryttani. How are you?' She speaks to everybody!" If someone asks why she looks different, Bryttani will say, "God made me this way because I'm special." Her parents let her handle herself because they know she can.

Bryttani is fortunate to have strong family support and an outgoing, confident personality. She's also had excellent medical care and support, as well as the benefit of being socialized from the time she was born. Attending PPEC nearly every day for her first five years helped Bryttani to become confident socially. "We've always taken her places with us," says Casey, from grocery stores to restaurants. "We're just in public a lot."

"She has a mind of her own and she tells it like it is," says Marcel. "It's shocking to me to be in a restaurant and have her grab the waitress's arm and say, 'Ma'am, please hurry, I'm allergic to waiting.'"

When Bryttani was in first grade last year, the school counselor was reading the children a story, the moral of which was that everyone's different. The teacher asked the class about being different and one boy shouted out, "Bryttani is different." The teacher feared the response would humiliate or hurt Bryttani. But the little boy followed by saying, "We love Bryttani!" And the whole class started chanting, "We love Bryttani! We love Bryttani! We love Bryttani!" and everybody gave her hugs.

"This was the regular class," says Casey, who is still touched by the children's response to her daughter. "They all love her," she says, adding that when Bryttani walks by kids lined up for a class, they give her high-fives.

Of course, not all children respond that way. When Bryttani meets new children, they sometimes shy away. "That's okay," she'll say, "you don't have to be shy."

Today, Bryttani has the perfect answer for anybody's questions, but as kids get older, they tease more because they move into that phase where they feel unsure of themselves. Bryttani surely will experience rejection as she gets older, and it will be painful. The question is how it will affect her self-esteem. Who will she see when she looks in the mirror: the special girl she's comfortable with now or a girl who can't make new friends? Will she be left outside the circle, and if so, how will she handle it?

"I just hope she continues to be so outgoing that nothing will get her down; that nothing will happen in the future; that nobody will come up to her and start picking on her, dragging her down," says Casey.

How Bryttani maintains self-esteem and deals with society will depend on several risk factors: medical, cognitive, functional, and psychosocial, says Dr. Kapp-Simon. The child and the family draw on resources that include the personality of the child, the family's mental health, socioeconomic factors, and how well the family handles stress. A child who is medically fragile and has severe physical and cognitive complications faces greater objective risk than a child whose medical and cognitive issues are minor. Similarly, a child with severe functional issues, such as learning disabilities and an inability to communicate, has a higher risk of poor adjustment.

"A child's inability to communicate affects how parents, teachers, and others relate to the child, which in turn impacts the child's ability to develop normal developmental skills, such as independence, social skills, and play," explains Dr. Kapp-Simon. Multiple surgeries and hospitalizations as well as differences in appearance contribute to the psychosocial risks a child faces. Children with chronic medical conditions have about twice the risk of poor adjustment that healthy children do, she says.

Two of the most crucial resources, however, are the child's own coping skills and self-esteem. A child who learns to cope well is better able to handle his or her fear or distress in a reasonable way. Positive coping may increase feelings of self-esteem. Stressful situations may be more difficult for some children, however. For example, a child who typically handles medical appointments well might feel anxious and afraid if the parent is visibly upset during an exam. Likewise, a fearful child can gain strength from a parent who is calm and reassuring during a medical appointment. "Based on their child's temperament, parents can develop strategies to help support the child and increase the risk of successful adaptation," says Dr. Kapp-Simon.

Temperament and self-esteem influence social skills, but many social skills can be taught. It's well established that children who look different from their peers have a harder time being accepted and initiating social interactions. Developing social coping strategies is an important step toward achieving positive social encounters.

"A preschool-aged child can learn to field questions about her appearance in a positive, friendly way," says Dr. Kapp-Simon, "learning how to talk about her difference just the way she would explain why she has brown hair instead of black hair, for example." Strategies for older children focus on eye contact, tone of voice, and using words to show interest in the topics discussed by a peer.

When Bryttani was just about five, her parents took her to a playground near their home. She befriended a little girl and they played together for about 20 minutes before the girl asked Bryttani why her left eye was closed. (Her parents had her take out her prosthetic eye before she played, so that she wouldn't lose it.) Bryttani responded, "Well, I don't have one. I only have one eye because I'm special. God made me that way," then turned around and started back up the ladder to the slide. The girl stood there for a minute thinking about it, shrugged her shoulders, and then followed Bryttani up the ladder. Later that evening,

Casey asked her daughter if that encounter had hurt her feelings, and Bryttani insisted that it hadn't.

"It would be okay if it had," explained Casey, "and it's okay to talk about it."

"She was only asking because she just wanted to know," Bryttani replied.

"Okay, as long as you know you can talk to me anytime about things like this."

Bryttani thought about it for a few seconds and then asked, "Mommy, did it hurt your feelings? Do you want to talk about it?"

BRYTTANI RECEIVES ALL HER specialized medical care at Children's Hospital of Philadelphia, commonly known as CHOP, which is a two-hour drive from her home in Milford, Delaware. Although Bryttani's cleft runs through her lip and palate, it also extends through the area where her nasal structure should be and to her eye, involving gaps in soft tissue and bone along the way. Because of this, she is considered to have a Tessier cleft. More complex than a cleft lip and palate, Tessier clefts can involve any combination of the lips, mouth, nose, cheeks, eyes, ears, and forehead. Tessier clefts are numbered from 0 to 14, depending on their location on the face. Bryttani appears to have Tessier clefts 0 and 14, which designate the midline of the face. What makes Bryttani's case more complex, however, is the fact that she's missing the majority of her nasal structure.

Cleft lip and palate is the most common craniofacial birth defect, affecting one in 700 children around the world, according to the Cleft Palate Foundation. Although a child could be born with just a cleft lip, usually the cleft involves the palate as well. Tessier clefts, on the other hand, are much less common, occurring in roughly one to five babies per 100,000 births. Clefts can run in families, but most of the time they occur spontaneously for no known reason. How and when a cleft is treated depends on its severity and type.

By age eight, Bryttani had already undergone six surgeries related to her craniofacial condition. Her cleft lip and soft palate were corrected. (Her hard palate will be fixed later, and she will have bone grafts and a jaw alignment to fix the cleft through her gum line.) She had two major ophthalmic surgeries. The first involved taking tissue from her buttocks to build up her eye socket so that it could better accommodate a prosthetic eye, which Bryttani has had since she was six months old. The second surgery was to insert a Jones tube, a device used to connect a functional tear duct to a nonfunctional or missing one. Ironically, Bryttani's left eye, which is missing, had a functional tear duct that her ophthalmic surgeon connected to her right eye, which was missing its tear duct.

Before her nasal passage is reconstructed, Bryttani needs orthodontic work on her upper jaw, or hard palate, which is split in two by the cleft. The hard-palate surgery will involve connecting the two sides with bone grafts and then aligning them into position. Bryttani's orthodontist is widening her upper jaw using an expander, a metal device fitted to the roof of her mouth and turned daily with a tiny key. The expansion will encourage her jaw to move forward and help to get her mouth structurally as close to "normal" as possible. That will have a big impact on her speech, says Casey. "It will cut down on, but not eliminate, the risk of her aspirating," she adds. "She has that risk constantly because she only has the one airway."

Once Bryttani is about 15, when she's finished growing and all her orthodontic work is done, Casey anticipates the nasal reconstruction will be performed. To create a nose for Bryttani, the plastic surgeon will cut a flap of skin from her forehead. One end of the flap will stay attached to her forehead and its original blood supply; the other end will be fashioned into a nose. The tissue will stay connected this way for about six weeks, after which the connection between the tissue and the forehead will be severed. The stub of tissue Bryttani was born with between her eyes also will be used to help create her nose.

If the surgery is attempted before Bryttani is finished growing, there's the risk of having to perform additional repairs to compensate for normal growth. Bryttani's plastic surgeon doesn't think she will breathe through her nose after her nasal reconstruction, but Casey is not so sure. Her daughter has surprised people before. "We never know with her," Casey laughs.

ALTHOUGH BRYTTANI'S APPEARANCE is secondary for Casey, she understands that the surgeries will be important for her confidence as she gets older. Marcel feels differently about his daughter. He says, "If it was my way, she would stay the way she is. To put her through all these surgeries…I hate to have her go through it. I think she's beautiful as she is."

Diana Sweeney, the parent liaison within the craniofacial center at CHOP, understands exactly how Marcel feels. Her son Dan had craniofacial surgery at CHOP as a boy, and she agonized about the decision. What finally helped her was looking beyond the moment and trying to imagine her son's future life. She couldn't allow herself to think about how the surgery would affect her. "I had to take myself out of the equation," she says.

Since then, she has worked with parents of children with craniofacial conditions and witnessed a lot of family dynamics. Fathers, she says, are usually very protective of their daughters with craniofacial conditions. Often, they'll say, "My daughter is beautiful. She doesn't need surgery." Sometimes, they'll feel terribly sorry for themselves, ashamed that this happened to them, and they can't move beyond that. Either way, Sweeney is the one who says, "Dad, it's not about you. This is all about your daughter." She works to get them to see past the surgery and to imagine their child going to prom, graduating from high school, going to college, getting married. She uses a progression of photographs of her own son to help illustrate her point, explaining to parents that she had similar feelings when she was faced with his surgery.

At CHOP, Sweeney serves as a link between the emotional and medical aspects of surgery. Parents often don't ask the doctors the "emotional" questions, she says, so instead, the parents hold the fear. She helps them make sense of their feelings and lets them know that it's okay to feel negative. "Part of my job is to tell them it's okay to hate it, to feel bad. You shouldn't like it," she says.

For Casey, showing her real feelings is a balancing act because of her daughter's intense fear of the hospital. "As Bryt's mother, I have to act as if everything is going to be okay," she says, while still being aware of the risks and the possibility that everything might not be okay. "I cannot let her even sense that I am afraid, nervous, or whatever. It's like I have to put a front on, as if I'm not worried and it's just another day, so that she'll be as calm as she can be and not be a nervous wreck or terrified."

Once Bryttani is wheeled into the operating room, Casey can let go, cry, and feel anxious. But until then, she puts up a strong front, at the same time worrying that her daughter might think she doesn't care because she's not showing her fear.

Sweeney says this type of response is typical. "I think that craniofacial parents sometimes don't want to acknowledge their own fear, so it is better not to discuss it at all!" she says. She acknowledges that there is a fine line about showing children fear but thinks that children Bryttani's age are old enough to handle some fear and that fear is inherent, not just with respect to surgery, but also in the larger context of life.

"I find my parents like to shield their children from any pain, no matter the source," says Sweeney. "This is totally understandable, but this world is not fear-free and they have to have a certain amount of exposure to fear in order to handle it in everyday life."

Children deserve age-appropriate information, nothing less and nothing more, along with a straightforward attitude, even if the parent doesn't feel very confident, says Sweeney. The fine line between sharing information and conveying concern has to be navigated thoughtfully. Surgery—and subsequent hospitalization—isn't a singular experience for the majority of children with craniofacial conditions, so parents can truly influence how a child reacts, not only to the current ordeal, but also to future ones.

"By telling them the truth about their upcoming surgery, sharing their fears and your own, a certain level of comfort can be reached through just plain honesty. I try to help my parents reach that level—not too much or too little but someplace that they are all somewhat comfortable," Sweeney says. "As parents, we transfer adult attitudes and fears to our children. I think this is totally wrong, as we must remember that they are children and really do not look at the world in quite the same way that we do. I think you can give too much information so as to scare them and also be so nonchalant that they don't trust you after they have had the surgical experience."

These are some of the issues that Sweeney deals with daily. She listens when a parent needs to talk, and she tells parents to call her anytime. She means it. Only once has a parent called her in the middle of the night, and she was happy to talk. When the situation warrants intervention, she refers the family to a social worker or psychologist.

To her knowledge, no one else does what she has been doing enthusiastically for 30 years. She also has been involved in the Children's Craniofacial Association for years, serving as a resource for parents, educating people, and creating awareness about craniofacial conditions. Giving back is her passion. When told she is amazing, she responds, "No, I'm so lucky."

CASEY AND MARCEL ARE striving for Bryttani to have the most normal life possible, especially because, in so many ways, Bryttani is just a typical kid. Sometimes she doesn't even understand that there are some things she can't do or that she might need accommodations to do some things. Her vision loss affects her hand-eye coordination, so she has trouble with balance. Still, she loves to dance and enjoyed taking ballet and tap lessons until it became too difficult to keep up with her classmates.

"We try to let her do as much as she wants and the things she wants, but it's hard when we have more safety issues to take into account than the typical parent," Casey says. Ordinarily, though, they let her at least try new things. Sometimes she'll excel at something, such as swimming, and love it. Other times, she finds that she can't do something and doesn't feel the way she thought she might. Then, Casey and Marcel are there to comfort her.

Bryttani has some vision in her right eye, but she is considered borderline legally blind. Casey fought since nearly day one for Bryttani to learn Braille in case she loses her eyesight completely. The problem was that, because she has some vision, the insurance company wouldn't pay for Braille lessons. Casey's philosophy is this: "She's going to have what she needs, even if I have to go sit on the White House steps, and if you're not going to help me, I'll find someone who will." After a year of pleading her case to Bryttani's visual therapist, and with the full support of her ophthalmologist at CHOP, Bryttani finally is receiving pre-Braille lessons.

CASEY WAS QUIET AND unassuming when she was younger. She had planned to become an elementary schoolteacher, with an emphasis on special education, but when her daughter was about a year old, the U.S. Department of Labor offered Casey free training as a certified nursing assistant. After working as a CNA for a month, she felt as though she'd found her niche. She studied to become a nurse, a profession she says she had never contemplated, "let alone one that I absolutely love." After finishing the RN program, she may enroll in a master's degree program, with the goal of perhaps becoming a nurse practitioner.

Although Casey, now 30, still appears waiflike, she's headstrong and assertive. She doesn't hold back her thoughts or mince words. "After I had Bryttani, I suddenly had a little person I needed to fight for; I mean really fight for, in some cases on a state level." Today, Casey is stronger than she ever was, but the stress of fighting with insurance companies, coordinating care, managing multiple medical appointments, and driving hours to get there can be overwhelming, mentally and physically. And there's no such thing as taking time for a real vacation; time off typically is used for surgeries.

Early in 2006, Casey came down with a serious kidney infection that resulted in kidney failure, landing her in the hospital. Her biggest fear is that something might happen that prevents her being there for her daughter. "That would be the only concern: Who would advocate for her as much as I do?" she asks.

After a rough day, or when Casey is feeling down, she simply looks at her inspiration, her daughter. *She's doing so well*, she thinks to herself. *She's been through so much and she's so strong.* At other times, she finds peace looking up at the night sky, each star a single truth, proof of endurance. When Casey pointed out the stars to Bryttani, she discovered that she couldn't see them because they're too far away. "The reality broke my heart because that's something I like to do," says Casey.

Casey and Marcel weren't sure what Bryttani could and couldn't see until recently. Playing in her mother's lap one day, she got a really close look at Casey's face. "Mommy, you have blue eyes!" she said. "It was the first time she's seen the color," says Casey. "It was a big moment for us. Now she wants a telescope so she can see the stars."

Casey has never been to a nightclub with girlfriends. She's never had her very own apartment, furnished with castaways from family members and flea-market finds. She didn't even have a wedding. Instead, she lives for her daughter's mischievous smile, intense curiosity, and funny way of pleading "Lord, help me; help me, please!" when she finds herself in a bit of a bind. Those things are her life's treasures.

When Casey and Marcel first learned of the extent of Bryttani's cleft before she was born, and shared the news with Marcel's parents, they told Casey and Marcel that things happen for a reason. God has a plan, they said, and Bryttani would be a blessing, no matter what was wrong. How right they were!

"God chose us for a reason. He gave us a very special gift," says Casey. She turns and asks her daughter, "How did I get such a special girl?"

Bryttani looks up at her mother's soft blue eyes and answers, "Because you're special, Mommy."

❀

CHAPTER 12

a posse ad esse: from possibility to actuality

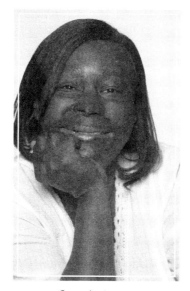

Gwen Arrington

*We began by imagining that we are giving to them;
we end by realizing that they have enriched us.*

—Pope John Paul II

WORLD WAR I INTRODUCED a great volume of facial injuries never seen before and gave surgeons a unique opportunity to devise new methods of treating them. Since then, physicians and researchers have been working to improve reconstructive surgery techniques and to develop new materials to replace damaged or deformed human tissue.

Recent advances in genetics research hold promise for helping us to understand and, it is hoped, prevent disfiguring birth defects. We look to science to help us live better, healthier lives, and we applaud the unwavering professionals who dedicate their careers to bringing sometimes seemingly outrageous ideas from possibility to actuality.

For at least three generations, many of the babies born into a particular family in Venezuela have had a peculiar appearance. The family's condition has no name. All have had eyes set very far apart and fatty tumors in the mid-face; some have had deformed eyelids and noses; and one family member, an adult woman, has part of her brain pushing through her left eye socket. That defect is called an encephalocele and can cause brain damage if not corrected.

"It's an ultra-rare disease that's never been categorized," says Dr. Christopher Gordon. "Out of forty-odd people, twenty-one are affected." He and his colleagues in Latin America have never seen anything quite like it.

Dr. Gordon, a plastic and reconstructive surgeon, is an assistant professor of plastic surgery at the University of Cincinnati and chair of surgery at Cincinnati Children's Hospital. He often travels to Latin American countries to perform pro bono facial reconstructive surgery. His trip to Venezuela in 2005 to treat several members of this family was at the request of a colleague, Dr. Leopoldo Landa, who practices there.

Many of the family members also have clefts that affect their eyes and eyelids. According to Dr. Gordon, the clefts exhibited by this family don't match the classical bony and soft-tissue clefts originally identified by Dr. Paul Tessier. Like their other symptoms, their clefts are rare.

Some family members underwent surgical correction years ago, but the results weren't good. Thanks to new surgical techniques, many of the family members were willing to try again. A few underwent facial bipartition, which involves halving the face vertically to advance the mid-face forward and realign the eyes. Others had a monobloc procedure, which also helps bring the forehead and the mid-face forward all at once.

There's little doubt that the Venezuelan family's syndrome has a genetic basis, so when Dr. Gordon was there last, he collected blood and tissue samples for genetic analysis. Because so many family members are affected, he was confident that his research team could come up with a short list of candidate genes and have the gene sequenced within three to four months. "We're entering the California gold rush of human genetics," says Dr. Gordon. "Find it, name it." Once they do, the syndrome will be named after the province where the family lives.

By identifying the gene or genes responsible for this family's deformities, Dr. Gordon hopes that future generations may be spared. Prevention and treatment might include in utero therapy or gene therapy for those who test positive for the mutation.

Currently, no gene therapy is available for craniofacial conditions. "We're teetering on the edge of being able to do it," says Dr. Gordon, but when a gene is inserted into the genome, the potential exists that it can disrupt another gene and cause another kind of problem. A pharmaceutical approach to treatment, rather than a gene therapy approach, may be more prudent.

In the United States, when 18-year-old Jesse Gelsinger died in 1999 after receiving gene therapy — less to treat his disease (ornithine transcarbamylase deficiency) than to help advance medical science — the practice hit the wall. Since then, researchers here and overseas have slowly been attempting gene therapy again and have actually celebrated a few successes. Dr. Gordon says researchers here are ready to get back on track.

GENE THERAPY MAY HOLD tremendous promise for people who need a section of bone replaced because of cancer, a congenital anomaly, or traumatic injury. Dr. Edward Schwarz, professor of orthopedics and of microbiology and immunology at the University of Rochester Medical Center in New York, is leading a team of researchers using gene therapy to convert a dead bone graft into living tissue in laboratory research.

Today, the standard treatment for someone with jaw cancer, for example, may involve transplanting autologous bone (bone that belongs to the patient). The problem is that the transplant procedure requires a separate surgery as well as the destruction of another bone. More often, a bone graft from a cadaver, called an allograft, is used. While the cadaveric bone provides necessary strength and structure, it tends to disintegrate as it ages because it's "dead."

"Our bones are subjected to microscopic fractures from everyday wear and tear," says Dr. Schwarz, "but are able to repair themselves constantly. However, when the bone is dead, it cannot heal itself, and those fractures begin to accumulate until finally, perhaps in ten years, the cadaveric bone graft fails."

Dr. Schwarz identified two key proteins, called RANKL and VEGF, necessary for bone regeneration. The genes responsible for those proteins were under-expressed in the cadaveric bone, which means enough of them weren't present to have a regenerative effect. By modifying a harmless virus to include the genes, Dr. Schwarz created what's called a viral paste, which is painted directly onto a bone graft during surgery. In his laboratory experiments, new blood vessels grew around and into the cadaveric bone graft. In other words, he was able to trick dead bone into thinking it was alive and part of the body's own tissue.

Dr. Schwarz believes that this technology, called rAAV-coated allograft, holds promise for craniofacial reconstructive surgery and has applied for grant funding for additional research. He also believes the technology has benefits over using stem cells. "We think that this approach overcomes the major limitations of stem cell technologies, which are: One, where do the cells in sufficient quantities come from? Two, how will they be maintained and quality-controlled at the hospital where they will be used? And, three, who will take responsibility for how they are applied to the carrier during reconstructive surgery?" In addition, the huge advance in rAAV-coated implants is that they can be reduced to an off-the-shelf product that can be shipped, stored, and handled, the same as the implants that are used today.

Science sometimes moves at glacial speed; some medical advances can take up to a decade to get from the laboratory to the bedside. It's hard to say how soon rAAV-coated implants might be available for people with craniofacial conditions, but Dr. Schwarz hopes to begin early human clinical trials soon and someday apply the technology to repair cartilage, which cannot regenerate itself, unlike bone. He says, "For reasons that have to do with the feasibility of performing a phase III clinical trial, our team, including the Musculoskeletal Transplant Foundation, is focusing on limb salvage allografting following resection of tumor in legs or arms as the first indication for rAAV-coated allografts. If this is successful, it is likely that the MTF would move quickly to supply rAAV-coated allografts for craniofacial reconstruction surgery."

EVERY RECONSTRUCTIVE SURGEON interviewed for this book said that the one thing that would make the job easier is availability of better materials to replace human tissue. Dr. Anthony Calabro Jr. is on the verge of introducing a new material that may have enormous impact on what surgeons can do for patients with facial damage. Currently, depending on the extent of the damage, the choices for repairing cartilage damaged by a birth defect, disease, or trauma are limited to two: a prosthesis or reconstruction using cartilage harvested from another part of the body, often the rib.

Dr. Calabro, a biochemist in the Biomedical Engineering Department at the Cleveland Clinic Lerner Research Institute, has been working on developing a novel hyaluronan–based hydrogel. The hydrogel is made from the same components as human cartilage, offering surgeons a limitless amount of material to mold into whatever they need.

One of the major advantages of the hydrogel is that its chemical composition can be modified to suit the surgical goal: filling a void, correcting a defect, coating a nonbiologic device or implant, or replacing an anatomic structure. For example, if a patient has lost his or her nose because of cancer, it is entirely conceivable that the scaffolding of the nose could be re-created using hydrogel. Tracheal reconstruction, which is a terribly difficult and complex procedure today, could be a comparative breeze using hydrogel. "Hydrogel could also be used to replace the vitreous humor in a detached retina. In the eye, hydrogel is completely transparent," Dr. Calabro says.

Working tirelessly in his laboratory, Dr. Calabro has re-created the natural macromolecular architecture of human cartilage by chemically modifying cartilage's natural components. The end result is a material that mechanically is very strong and versatile. Hydrogel can be used to replace not only missing cartilage, but also a variety of soft tissues.

"The material is built on the same molecules as natural human cartilage. It's a complicated, elegant interplay using carbohydrates, which give the material its properties, without the proteins that would cause the body to break it down," says Dr. Calabro. Because the carbohydrates used in the formula are found throughout the body, the chances of the body rejecting the material as foreign are slim.

Developing a material that won't cause immune issues over the long term is crucial. In addition, the hydrogel must be biocompatible, nontoxic, and noninflammatory, and it must be able to be integrated into existing and newly formed tissue structures. This property is crucial in craniofacial reconstruction, because too often replacement tissues don't want to stay put, he says. They want to migrate.

So far, the results of animal studies have shown promise. "Hydrogel is an inert scaffolding material. It's hard to imagine that the immune system won't tolerate it," notes Dr. Calabro, whose next step is to seek approval from the U.S. Food and Drug Administration to begin testing hydrogel in humans.

IN 2004, A TEAM IN GERMANY used a technique called tissue engineering to create a replacement jaw for a 56-year-old man who had lost his lower jaw to squamous cell cancer. His head and neck area also had been damaged from radiation treatment. Using three-dimensional CT and computer-aided design technology, a model of the patient's head was created. Next, a titanium-mesh scaffold of his jaw was created; filled with hydroxyapatite, bone-inducing protein, and bone marrow; and then implanted into the patient's latissimus dorsi muscle, which runs underneath the arm, along the side of the back, and across the lumbar region.

Seven weeks later, the regenerated jaw was removed, along with some of the dorsi muscle that contained its blood supply, and transplanted to the man's face. Four weeks later, the patient ate bread and sausages, the first solid food he'd been able to eat in nine years. Although the long-term effects of this experimental procedure won't be known for several years, at least in the short run one can assume the patient's quality of life improved dramatically.

BROTHERS CHARLES VACANTI, head of anesthesiology at Brigham and Women's Hospital, and Joseph Vacanti, a pediatric surgeon at Massachusetts General Hospital, along with Dr. Robert Langer, professor of chemical and biomedical engineering at Massachusetts Institute of Technology, are pioneers in tissue engineering. In 1997, they implanted human cartilage on the back of a mouse and grew an ear — one of the most difficult human structures to re-create. The experiment stemmed from their desire to advance tissue engineering to the point of creating replacement organs, so that no one would have to die while waiting for a donor organ.

The idea came to Dr. Joseph Vacanti in 1986 while he was vacationing at Cape Cod. Wading in shallow water, he was inspired by the intricate branching networks of seaweed and got the idea to create bio-degradable scaffolding that could be filled with cells, which would then grow and fill the structure.

Since then, Dr. Charles Vacanti has fashioned a new thumb for a patient, and his brother has created skin replacement tissue for burn vic-tims. Both now are working on a trial involving patients who have had intervertebral discs removed. Traditional repair would involve implant-ing spacers made from titanium; instead, the brothers are planning to implant autologous stem cells into biodegradable scaffolding. Because the cells come from the person's own body, they are biocompatible and don't pose the same risk of rejection as cells from donors.

Tissue engineering technology is novel, and few centers in the world are involved in its research. One of the main benefits of perfecting the technology is the solution to the problem of the availability of "parts."

MORE THAN A DECADE AGO, Dr. Dario Fauza, a pediatric surgeon at Children's Hospital in Boston, worked on a baby who was born with a hole in his chest wall — a hole so large that the baby's heart was out-side his body. He and his team tried everything they could to patch the hole, but the right material simply didn't exist. In adults, surgeons often can borrow tissue from other parts of the body. Newborns, how-ever, don't have enough extra tissue for this purpose, and transplant-ing tissue isn't an option for two reasons, explains Dr. Fauza: First, at least for now, unlike whole organs (such as the liver, with the big blood vessels that feed it), it is virtually impossible to preserve living tissue outside the body for many hours; and second, there is a universal lack of donors. The baby, who was otherwise healthy, expectedly died from infection.

Since then, Dr. Fauza has committed himself to creating tissue for his youngest patients while gestation is still ongoing, using fetal cells. This way, the engineered tissue is available for implantation at birth or even in the womb. In research studies involving large-animal models, he has used the cells to create patches for neonatal repair of hernias in the diaphragm, a relatively common birth defect in human babies, and to repair tracheal defects in utero. In both scenarios, the defects are life-threatening; hence his immediate focus. The implications of this new technology for babies born with craniofacial problems are tremendous.

"I think there's overlap with what we're doing," says Dr. Fauza, who now is working on a project to treat cleft palate using fetal cell–based tissue engineering. Many craniofacial problems are identified before birth, so a "fix" could be prepared before the baby is born and applied soon after birth, later, or, depending on the problem, possibly even before he or she is born. Tissue engineering may obviate the traditional need for waiting until a child has finished growing before beginning certain craniofacial repairs. An early repair can offer a better outcome for many congenital anomalies, he says, so perhaps this also will be the case for craniofacial anomalies once this technology matures.

Dr. Fauza often uses fetal cells taken from amniotic fluid, which is routinely collected from many women sometime around the 16th week of pregnancy to test for chromosomal disorders. Fetal cells also are available from the fetus itself, the placenta, and umbilical cord blood, but taking them from amniotic fluid is less invasive and causes no additional risk to the mother or fetus. Because the cells are easy to isolate from the amniotic fluid, a spoonful of fluid is all that is needed.

For his research, Dr. Fauza uses a particular type of fetal cell called a mesenchymal stem cell. Although mesenchymal stem cells have only about one-third the capabilities of embryonic stem cells, they are unspecialized and can generate many types of tissue.

"Although these cells are not as powerful as embryonic cells because they cannot be turned into anything, they can be turned into most anything we need for surgical repair," he says. "I don't necessarily want to make a new eye or tongue; typically, just bone, cartilage, muscle, and tendon. I can do a lot with that."

The main benefit of using these mesenchymal cells is that nothing new is being created. Dr. Fauza says, "Unlike therapeutic cloning, in which you typically have to take the nucleus of a cell from a patient, put it in an egg, and try to make an embryo, and then take the embryonic stem cells, we're not creating anything. These cells are already floating in the amniotic fluid. They'll be thrown out when the baby is born. I don't see any ethical objection."

Another benefit is that fetal cells grow quickly, he says. The cells are easily coaxed into doing what the researchers want. Because they are immunologically immature and trigger a low rejection response, one conceivably could take fetal cells from the amniotic fluid of one pregnancy and use them on a baby in a different pregnancy. "Ideally, you'd use cells from the same baby, because then you have a zero risk of rejection," says Dr. Fauza.

Yet another benefit is timing. He explains, "We can engineer the tissue while the baby is gestating. You can start the rebuilding process even before birth, possibly." This is exactly how Dr. Fauza envisions the hernia patch working in babies. When a congenital diaphragmatic hernia is identified in a fetus through an ultrasound, the next step would be to collect amniotic fluid, from which mesenchymal cells are isolated. The cells would then be expanded and used to create a tendon patch that is ready and waiting for the baby to be born. Once born, the baby would undergo surgery to correct the hernia.

The only downside, as Dr. Fauza sees it, is the possibility that the long-term results won't be as promising as expected. "We have good short- to mid-term data, but we don't know the long term," he says. Still, he's enthusiastic about the possibilities.

Fetal cells can be stored for future use, so they could be helpful to babies who need repairs as they grow and could also conceivably be helpful throughout life, he says. For example, the Teflon patches now used to repair hernias in infants pull out and rupture over time. (A human diaphragm more than quadruples in size from birth to adulthood.) Theoretically, patches engineered from fetal cells grow and remodel as the child does. In research studies in large animals mimicking similar growth, Dr. Fauza's team found that the tendon patches held up without any problem.

"We're very close to the first human trial," he says. The study will enroll 20 pregnant women who are known to be carrying babies with hernias. Amniotic fluid will be collected from each of the mothers, and a customized tendon patch will be created and ready for the babies when they're born.

The first step is getting approval from the FDA. Because the technology is so new, the field must be redefined, which may complicate the approval process. "In one way, it's cell-based therapy; in another way, it's biologic therapy because we're seeding cells onto a biological scaffold," he explains. Although the process for FDA approval may be time-consuming and sometimes frustrating for all parties, the sense is that the eventual outcome will be well worth it. Says Dr. Fauza, "You have to blaze the trail."

TISSUE ENGINEERING COMBINES principles of engineering and developmental biology to give the body the help it needs to repair or regenerate damaged tissue, says Dr. Gordana Vunjak-Novakovic, professor of biomedical engineering at Columbia University in New York City. Tissue engineering works by inserting specialized cells into a biologic scaffold and guiding them toward specific tissue outcomes. The scaffold or support structure is designed to mimic the structure of normal tissue so that the cells encounter an environment that appears familiar. The tissue is exposed to all the factors it needs to function properly, such as nutrients, growth factors, and vitamins, as well as oxygen and physical stimuli. "If the conditions are right, the cells will respond to this environment in the right way. The cell is the builder of the tissue, and we're just assisting the cell in this process," says Dr. Vunjak-Novakovic.

Tissue engineered in a patient's own body, particularly from a patient's own cells, is preferable to donated tissue because it doesn't involve the risk of rejection. Likewise, natural tissues or those engineered using inert materials are preferred over artificial materials. Sometimes the body will treat the artificial material as a foreign invader and will attack it, surrounding it with scar tissue, absorbing it, or attempting to push it out. This forces the surgeon and the patient to come up with another solution.

To avoid those situations, says Dr. George Muschler, orthopedic surgeon and director of the Bone Biology Laboratory at Cleveland Clinic, surgeons rely on a variety of artificial materials, such as biocompatible polymers or plastics, ceramics, or hydrogels, to get the results they want. "The goal is generally to use a material that can allow growth and remodeling of tissue in the region of the implant. In this case, bone will not only grow into void spaces in the material, but the material may also resorb, allowing the bone to change and fill more of the void over time," he says. "Alternatively, one could consider inert materials that do not resorb. In this case, the material must allow intimate attachment through ingrowth of local bone but may persist over time to provide normal function and normal appearance."

Dr. Muschler, who also co-directs the Center for Tissue Engineering, a multi-institution collaboration, defines tissue engineering as "any process where we're trying to get tissue that we want where we want it and keep it there." Tissue engineering strategies include preserving, augmenting, repairing, replacing, or regenerating existing tissue.

Bone marrow is a source of cells that can make a wide variety of tissues. "There are cells in bone marrow that can make blood tissue, nerve tissue, liver tissue, muscle, fat, tendon, ligaments, bone, and cartilage. You can even make dermal tissue, the tissue underneath the surface of your skin, though not epidermis [the tissue that covers the surface of your skin]," he explains. By isolating and transplanting specific cells from one or more sources, such as bone marrow and skin, researchers hope to learn how to direct cells to grow into specific desired tissues (such as cartilage, muscle, or bone) after they are transplanted. Some scientists are working to develop these tissues outside the body first, even before they are transplanted.

"That's one of the areas that's perhaps the most fascinating to people inside and outside of the medical field; the complexity and even the clinical need for this approach can be sometimes overstated," says Dr. Muschler.

Prior to joining Columbia, Dr. Vunjak-Novakovic collaborated with tissue engineering pioneer Robert Langer and shifted her interest from chemical engineering to bioengineering. She has received more than $5 million in new research grants for craniofacial and cardiac tissue engineering, two areas that are among her research specialties. Now she is concentrating on building functional tissues, using embryonic and adult human stem cells, biomaterials, and bioreactors.

"Stem cells are original or source cells. They're undecided about where to go," she explains. Stem cells can do two things: They can renew or maintain themselves, or they can evolve into different cell types. Although adult stem cells are not as versatile as embryonic stem cells, they do have tremendous abilities to renew themselves, even in the elderly or people who are seriously ill. "The cartilage and bone in an 80-year-old is relatively useless because of its age," says Dr. Vunjak-Novakovic, but if you take the stem cells from that person, you may be able to create functional tissue.

An ongoing project for Dr. Vunjak-Novakovic is re-creating one of the most challenging tissues in the body: the temporomandibular joint, which is the hinge that connects the lower jaw to the temporal bone of the skull. A worn temporomandibular joint is very painful, and a good solution to the problem doesn't yet exist. Rather than attempting to repair or replace missing tissue, what if we could somehow encourage our bodies to renew tissue on their own?

"People have always been enthralled with the fact that if you're an amphibian and your limb is cut off, you'll regrow it," says Dr. Muschler. "And that includes skin, muscle, tendons, ligaments, blood vessels, and nerves. We usually think it's pretty good to be human, but this is one case where amphibians have us beat. Why is this so? Has evolution somehow resulted in the loss of this biologic potential in higher animals? Or has evolution added new mechanisms of healing, such as more rapid scar formation, that may overwhelm or inhibit a natural healing potential we still have and which might be unlocked again? This is an open question and the subject of a lot of research."

Dr. Muschler explains, "When we're young, even we humans, we don't form scars; rather, we regenerate tissues. If a baby undergoes surgery inside the uterus, he or she is born without a scar. If a baby is injured or undergoes surgery soon after birth, he or she won't scar. The tissue regenerates and repairs. However, as we age, we increasingly form scar tissue, rather than regenerate tissue. Within a few months or a year of birth, the scars we form become permanent marks that chronicle major repair events in our lives."

Scarring is, of course, very important for our survival, says Dr. Muschler. For example, if you cut yourself deeply, your body works hard to stem the flow of blood and close the wound with thick, fibrous scar tissue. In the future, we might not only control the bleeding and heal the wound but also try to modulate the way in which a scar forms to unmask an innate ability to regenerate tissue.

Although key strides have been made in many clinical settings, with bone marrow transplantation, bone grafting, treatment of burns, and regeneration of whole organs or joints, the technology is not yet ready for prime time. Much of the research is still either in the laboratory or in the translational stage—meaning that it is gearing up to be tested in humans. "Is it five years? Is it ten years?" asks Dr. Vunjak-Novakovic. "I don't know; you make progress, and you hit an obstacle and it takes you back three years. I'm convinced we're getting there. It's in the foreseeable future."

Medical advances aren't just about disease prevention and treatment, she says, but about quality of life, especially when a medical problem, such as a badly disfigured face, affects a person's emotional well-being. In those cases, finding a medical solution is valuable. "It's not a life-threatening situation in many cases, but it changes the whole life of a person," she says. "It's really important."

❈

CHAPTER 13

living between worlds

I celebrate myself, and sing myself.

—Walt Whitman, "Song of Myself"

THE DAY WAS BALMY, typical mid-May weather in northeast Ohio—warm in the sun but still cool enough for a jacket and long pants. Gwen Arrington had stopped by her parents' house on her way home from work to pick up her daughter, Al-Lexis, who was about 18 months old. Gwen's parents watched their granddaughter during the day when Gwen, then 22, was working. While she was at her folks' house, her father asked her to leave Lexis (as she was called) and pick her up later. Her father, a quiet, stoic man, had never done that before, but after he insisted two more times that the baby should stay, Gwen consented, thinking that maybe he just wanted to spend a little more time with Lexis and this was his way of asking.

With the sun heading into the western sky, the temperature was dropping quickly. Gwen hadn't worn a coat that day, so she borrowed a neighbor's jacket to wear for the bus ride home. The men's jacket, made of heavy wool, was too big for Gwen's small frame, but she took it and left, leaving her daughter behind. The ride home seemed long without her daughter sitting next to her, chattering away, although the only intelligible words she knew then were "mama" and "dada." Later, Gwen would thank God that Lexis hadn't been with her.

When Gwen arrived home, she could smell the gas as she was walking up the driveway. *There's a gas leak,* she thought. Her husband, Al, was probably upstairs sleeping. After working all day, he'd often come home and take a nap. Once he was asleep, he wasn't easy to wake up and if he'd been sleeping in a houseful of leaking gas, it would be even harder to rouse him. She yanked open the side door and inhaled against her will — the stench! The air was so thick with gas, a sudden idea could have ignited it.

Knowing that she had to get to him right away, she sprang up the stairs and headed for the bedroom. "Al! Get up!" she cried. The moment he opened his eyes, Gwen started for the door. But Al was still foggy from sleep and didn't notice the smell of gas in the house, the smell that Gwen was gagging on. He reached over to the bedside table and grabbed a cigarette. Putting it to his lips, he struck the lighter, and his right arm went up in flames. In less than an instant, the bedroom was engulfed in a blue ball. Al lost sight of Gwen, just as he was knocked to the floor. "Every time I tried to get up, it was like someone was holding me there," he says.

The flames were as nimble as a gymnast, leaping and flipping from wall to wall. The air was on fire.

Gwen managed to make it to the upstairs hallway, which was a blue flame. All she could think about was something she'd learned in junior high school chemistry class: A blue flame is the hottest point on a Bunsen burner. "It's funny what you remember," she says. At the top of the stairs, she, too, was knocked to the floor. She just needed to get down the stairs and through the front door.

Gwen scrambled to get up, but three more times she was knocked back to the floor. Finally, she gave up. *Oh my God, I'm going to die,* she thought. And then her daughter's face flashed in front of her, and she cried, "God, I can't go!" Then, as though she were being lifted, she was able to stand and get down the stairs. She grabbed the door handle and pushed, but the door wouldn't open. She pushed harder. Nothing. Angrily, she kicked the door with all her strength, but it still didn't budge. She stood quietly and prayed, "God, please help me." And then she remembered that the door pulled open. She turned the handle and stumbled out.

The crowd that had gathered around the burning house watched in horror as a woman, who was still smoking from being on fire, staggered down the driveway.

Gwen looked around. She wondered where Al was. She wondered why people were staring at her. And where was the help? *I was trapped in there for so long*, she thought. There was no sign of fire trucks or ambulances, not even a siren's cry in the distance. Reasoning that she had better call for help, Gwen started walking to the corner pay phone. She was waiting for the light to cross the street when two men retrieved her and brought her back. *Great! I finally make it down the street, and you're going to take me back to where I came from!* she thought. *Nobody was there to help me; that's why I came here!* But she was too much in shock to argue, so she allowed herself to be returned home.

By that time, the paramedics had arrived. Gwen sat down in a chair, and a neighbor poured cold water on her from a green bowl. Still there was no sign of Al, which meant he was trapped inside the house. The firefighters hoisted a ladder against the front of the house and were preparing to go in when a tremendous explosion rocked the entire street. The front of the house blew off, sending the ladder flying backward.

When the house exploded, Al was sure he was going to die. Through the flames and the smoke, he couldn't find the stairs. He couldn't find the door. He couldn't find a way out. And he knew that if the fire didn't kill him, the smoke would. He cried for help, and that's when the firefighters rescued him — he had unwittingly made it downstairs to the door. Al sat on the lawn, in shock, as the rescue workers doused him with water. A woman he didn't recognize walked toward him. He thought it odd that she had just one spot of hair on top of her head.

The paramedics took Gwen away in an ambulance, just as a second ambulance was transporting Al to the hospital. He was in agony, but he'd have to wait until he got to the hospital before he could be given anything for pain. Al's body felt as though it was still on fire, and no amount of writhing or yelling was going to make the pain go away. His flesh was melting, turning to liquid all over the gurney. On the way to the hospital, Al's screams competed with the blare of the ambulance siren. The young paramedic sitting with him cried.

Gwen suffered third- and fourth-degree burns over 28 percent of her body, mainly her face and hands. Her husband had first- and second-degree burns on 48 percent of his body, mostly on his torso. Both were in critical condition when they arrived at MetroHealth Medical Center in Cleveland. When their respective parents arrived at the hospital, they were told to see Gwen and Al right away because the medical staff wasn't sure they'd make it through the night.

THE SKIN, WHICH IS composed of three layers, essentially has two main functions: to protect the body from foreign invasion and to regulate body temperature. The top layer, called the epidermis, acts as a protective sheath, like paint on a car. Beneath it is the dermis, which is a layer of tough, rubbery connective tissue designed to protect the body from violent insults. The dermis houses blood vessels, hair follicles, and glands, as well as nerve endings so that the skin is sensitive enough to know what it should keep out, such as sharp knives and open flame. Deep beneath the dermis is a third, fatty layer, which offers yet another measure of protection.

Fire does to skin, tissue, muscle, and bone what it does to everything else in its path: consumes it wholesale. First-degree burns involve just the epidermis and feel like a sunburn. Second-degree burns, which involve the epidermis and part of the dermis, cause blisters and swollen, oozing wounds, as well as indescribable pain. People who know will tell you that burns are the most painful injury one can endure. To heal burns and prevent infection, the wounds must be debrided, or scraped clean, daily. Dead tissue is removed from the wounds using enzymes, high-powered water, or surgical tools. No method is painless.

Third- and fourth-degree burns, also known as full-thickness burns, affect all the layers of the skin, the nerves, blood vessels, and muscle. A fourth-degree burn will char bone. Severe scarring, amputation, and loss of function are real risks. Almost a third of Gwen's body was burned deeply. She would learn later that the wool jacket she'd borrowed that day saved her upper body from being ravaged by the flames and her leather loafers protected her toes. Denim, however, not only doesn't offer much protection from fire, but it also holds in the heat, especially if it is tight-fitting. Gwen's jeans, combined with her choice of socks — nylon knee-highs that fused with her flesh — resulted in profound burns to her legs. Her nail polish, acting as an accelerant, sent flames shooting from her fingertips and left her with little more than charred sticks for fingers. The only good thing about third- and fourth-degree burns is that there's little to no pain at first, because the nerves have been destroyed.

In the hospital, Gwen and Al were in rooms next to each other. In a large window across the hall, Al could see the reflection of a red light coming from Gwen's room. The light came from the pulse oximetry device clipped to the end of Gwen's big toe. Al watched the light as though it were his wife's heartbeat. As long as that red light was glowing, he knew Gwen was alive.

WEEKS WENT BY BEFORE Gwen emerged from critical care; finally, it was safe for doctors to attend to her badly damaged hands. The smell of the fire clung to what was left of her ashen fingers. On Gwen's left hand, surgeons amputated her pinkie finger and index finger down to the last joint, and the two fingers in between to the joint closest to the fingernail. The tip of her thumb also was amputated. All four fingers on her right hand were amputated at the first joint, just below the nail. Only her right thumb remained intact. Skin grafts taken from her buttocks were used to repair the top and inside of her left hand and the fingers on her right hand. As a result, Gwen wouldn't eat with her hands for a long time afterward. She laughs about it now, but says her hands felt dirty to her. "That's something you can't wash away!" she says, giving a soulful laugh.

All this time, Gwen did not have a clear idea of the extent of her injuries. The only injuries she knew about were the ones she could see — the injuries to her hands. She still wasn't experiencing much pain, except for the spots on her buttocks where the skin grafts were taken. The hospital staff and her family members didn't bat an eye when they looked at her. There simply were no signals that would have prompted her to think anything else was wrong. Then one day, she climbed out of her hospital bed to use the bathroom and noticed the mirror. Realizing that she hadn't seen herself for weeks, she took a look. From down the hall, patients, visitors, and staff heard the sound of a woman wailing.

Al was released from the hospital within a month. He stayed with his parents until he'd made arrangements for another place to live. In the meantime, Lexis stayed with Gwen's parents. For a while, Al saw a psychiatrist to help him with his guilt. He would blame himself for the accident for years, often questioning why Gwen had to bear the brunt of the injuries. "I have to learn how to forgive myself," he says.

Eight weeks after the fire, Gwen emerged from the hospital. She went to live with her parents because she needed so much care. She needed intensive outpatient therapy, which would last well over a year, to help her take care of her wounds, learn to walk again, and use her hands. The last time she had used her hands was to escape from a burning house. It would be a year and a half before she would use them again. Until then, Gwen's mother took complete care of her. Gwen was racked with guilt. "It was like being a baby all over again. I felt like she'd done this once; why does she have to do it again?" she says. "I just thought it was so unfair to her."

Lexis, who would turn two the following month, now was talking in sentences. Although she had been okay when she had visited her mother in the hospital, she felt differently when Gwen was back home. In fact, she was horrified. "My mommy is in the hospital," she'd say to Gwen. "You're not my mommy." Lexis carried a photograph of Gwen at 14. She'd hold it up, point to the girl in the photo, and say, "This is my mommy."

Gwen's father tried to soothe his granddaughter and encouraged her to kiss her mother, but Lexis would have no part of it. "He meant well, but she would just scream. She didn't want to be in the same room with me," laments Gwen.

In an instant, Gwen's entire life had changed. She lost her appearance and her ability to function independently. She lost her job and the place she called home, along with everything she owned. She had no money and no health insurance. Her only child was afraid of her, and her future held only one certainty: multiple surgeries.

Suicide seemed a good option, but she couldn't use her hands to kill herself. Says Gwen, "I found that so ironic, thinking, 'Great! I have to ask for help with that!'"

While she was still in the hospital, the staff had arranged for psychological therapy, but Gwen found it more annoying than helpful. The sessions stirred up too many emotions, and there was never enough time to resolve them. Even on days when she felt good, she'd leave the therapy sessions feeling awful. An hour just wasn't long enough to start and finish an emotional journey. "I was left on my own to pull myself together just so I could walk out of there," she says.

Other burn survivors visited Gwen in the hospital, but none of them looked the way she did. Everyone looked normal to her — no one else had severe burn injuries to the face — and she knew she was far from normal. The only satisfaction she got was from going to support groups and helping others. If the others looked at Gwen and thought *At least I'm not burned as badly as she is,* and that helped them move forward, that was okay with her. "I did want to be there for someone else," she says.

The unavailability of help would force Gwen to deal on her own with her despair, hopelessness, anger, and thoughts of suicide. Somehow, she would have to find a way. Her life depended on it.

BURN SURVIVORS NEED TO wear pressure garments, essentially around-the-clock for a year or more, to prevent scar tissue from developing. In Gwen's case, she was outfitted in pressure garments that covered her entire head — the face mask had holes for her eyes, nose, mouth, and ears — as well as her body, legs, and hands. She looked like a mummy. The long looks, people tripping over their own feet staring at her, and the double takes felt very personal. Gwen found herself staying indoors as much as possible. She'd go out for her therapy appointments, but if her mother needed to stop at a store on the way home, Gwen usually waited in the car.

Once, on the way back from an appointment, her mother stopped at a gas station. Gwen was reclining in the backseat, her head propped up on the rear door, watching everything going on from the eyeholes in her face mask. Suddenly, commotion erupted because the gas station clerk had spotted her and thought she was going to rob them.

If she did go to a grocery store, she'd go only with her best friend. "Karla would say, 'Take a picture! It lasts longer!' That made me feel good," says Gwen, who was feeling so low, she couldn't stick up for herself. That she had someone to protect and defend her was a gift.

The reaction of strangers was difficult, but the reaction of her daughter was unbearable. When Gwen moved out of her parents' home, Lexis stayed behind. At one point, Lexis felt comfortable enough to visit during the daytime but wanted to go back to her grandparents' home in the evening. Eventually, Lexis would stay entire weekends with her parents. She was getting more and more comfortable being in the same room with her mother, as long as Gwen didn't get too close. Finally, she moved back into her own house, which was an emotional relief for Gwen, as well as a big help. Gwen needed another pair of hands around the house, even if they did belong to a toddler.

Before long, Lexis became a little mother to Gwen, making sure she took her "itch pills" (as burns heal, they itch terribly) and looking out for her general well-being. One day, Lexis called home from her grandparents' house and asked her mother whether she'd eaten. When Gwen replied that she hadn't, Lexis asked to speak to her uncle, who was there visiting. Says Gwen, "The next thing I knew, my brother-in-law was in the kitchen, cooking me something to eat!"

Lexis also developed an uncanny knack of knowing what Gwen was thinking and feeling. Once, when Gwen was just sitting quietly crying, two-year-old Lexis approached her and said, "It's okay, Mommy. You're beautiful to me." For all Lexis knew, Gwen says, she could have been crying because she couldn't pay a bill, but it just so happens that she was crying because she felt so ugly.

Her mother's injuries affected Lexis in an unexpected way. When she was five, she went through a phase of stealing things from stores and friends' houses. Reasoning with her didn't work, nor did spanking her. Gwen and Al took her to the police station, hoping to scare her straight, but Lexis wasn't giving up her life of crime that easily. Then her parents considered what she was stealing: lipstick, perfume, makeup, rings, earrings—all things associated with beauty. When they confronted her, they discovered that Lexis felt she could prevent her appearance being taken from her by having makeup and trinkets. Her parents assured her that what had happened to Gwen probably wouldn't happen to her and that those things couldn't prevent an accident anyway. Finally, Lexis felt more secure and stopped stealing.

Years later, Gwen would feel that she had deprived Lexis of her childhood. Her daughter, barely two at the time of the accident, was thrust into a situation that required her to be mature well beyond her age. She was trying to be so responsible, watching out for her mother, helping to take care of her. She grew up too fast. But it wasn't only Lexis; Gwen felt she had placed many people in difficult positions.

GWEN HAD BEEN WORKING since she was a teen—sometimes two jobs, just for the extra cash. Before the accident, she had worked as an office manager for an alarm company and had a second job at a store. Of course, since the accident, neither she nor Al had been working and the family was struggling. All their possessions were lost in the fire, except for a few photographs and, oddly enough, Gwen's old Tupperware containers and their contents: flour, sugar, and coffee. She and her husband had to rebuild from the ground up, for themselves and for their young daughter.

Almost fully covered in pressure garments, Gwen walked into the Social Security office in Cleveland with her mother, hoping to apply for Social Security income because of her disability. It was an uphill battle right away, says Gwen. First, the office clerk was adamant that Gwen read and sign the papers, even though it was obvious that she couldn't. At the time, only her right thumb worked. Next, the worker denied her disability, saying that she didn't have enough earned-income credit, even though she'd been working since she was 16. Gwen's mother took over at that point. Reading through all the paperwork, she discovered that Gwen actually had two more credits than she needed.

"I can see you read a lot," the clerk said to Gwen's mother.

"That's what you have to do when people don't do their jobs," she fired back.

The clerk then told Gwen she would have to be examined by a state doctor to establish eligibility. By the time Gwen and her mother left the Social Security office, they were at wit's end. At home, Gwen called the 800 number for Social Security and spoke with a friendly voice from the state of Maryland, who informed her that she need only sign medical release forms. She even mailed the forms to Gwen. There was no reason to see a state doctor. It took a person three states away to help Gwen get her disability income.

Not content with doing nothing, Gwen decided that her best course of action would be to go back to school. It had been roughly three years since the fire, and "I wasn't doing anything else, just waiting for surgeries," she says. Besides, she knew that because of her facial scarring, people were going to discriminate against her and she wanted to make it as hard as possible for them to do so. She went to the Ohio Bureau of Vocational Rehabilitation and was told that she would have to take out student loans. Al hadn't been back to work very long and Gwen hadn't worked for three years. Al's paycheck and her disability payments barely kept food on the table. There was no way she could take out student loans. As Gwen walked out of the Ohio BVR office, she felt left behind, like scuff marks on a floor.

"IT'S LIKE LIVING BETWEEN worlds," says Gwen, explaining that you accept people's comments and try to explain human ignorance to your friends and family, who see you as normal, without scars. When she's out in public, she forgets that she looks different until someone reminds her with a comment, an insult, or an extended stare. It's the loss of anonymity and the ability to blend in that she misses the most. To go unnoticed, to move through a crowd like the wind...

"From time to time, I wish I was normal. I move along, but I wish I was normal," says Gwen. "I don't want to cause second looks."

After the fire, Gwen met with a plastic surgeon who was honest and straightforward, two qualities that anyone who is disfigured can appreciate. He told her to bring in photos of herself before the accident, but he cautioned that he would not be able to make her look like that again. He would, however, do the best he could.

The trouble with burns is the scar tissue, even with pressure garments. Because Gwen's injuries were so deep and she had so much scar tissue, not much reconstructive surgery could be done for her. Most of her prior surgeries involved skin grafts. When a face needs to be patched with skin, the patch isn't one large sheet; rather, it is little pieces placed next to and over each other, leaving seams that linger. Gwen's plastic surgeon concentrated on smoothing out the seams on her face from all the skin grafts.

The other trouble with burns is that for years after an injury, the scar tissue continues to tighten, causing functional problems as well as deformity. Most of Gwen's surgeries have been done to release the scar tissue that tightens and pulls underneath her facial skin and down into her neck. Several times, her mouth began to close and surgery was needed to cut the corners to open it. She also has had surgeries to release the tissue in what's left of her fingers so that she can continue to use her hands. Eventually, though, the scar tissue tightens again.

The last time Gwen found herself in a surgical prep room — she'd had more than 30 surgeries by that point — she had reached her limit. With a pillow under her head and a sheet pulled over her, the smell of the hospital engulfed her. It stank of unfairness. The smell filled her lungs, the way the gas had 15 years before. She wanted to run, find the door, and make her way outside to safety. The overhead lights felt hot on her skin and the nurses' chatter grew louder until it buzzed inside her head. Gwen clutched the bed rails to steady her trembling hands and then screamed as she never had before.

Barbara Kammerer Quayle is a burn survivor who has worked tirelessly since her accident to help people with facial burns heal after they leave the hospital. She pioneered the School Reentry Program for burn-injured children and Behavioral and Enhancement Skill Tools (BEST) to benefit community reentry for burn survivors. She authored *THE BOOK of Image Enhancement for Burn Survivors*: *A common-sense approach to creating your BEST image* and participates in an accompanying how-to video and CD. She coordinates the BEST program for the Phoenix Society for Burn Survivors, a national nonprofit organization, and conducts BEST program workshops at burn centers in the United States and internationally to train staff in the "coaching" skills to assist their patients and families.

Years earlier, Kammerer Quayle was a passenger in a car stopped at a stoplight. The car behind hers didn't stop, exploding the gas tank as it rear-ended the car she was in. She was rescued by a passerby and was transported to the UC Irvine Medical Center in California, where she spent more than two months. She lost the fingers on her right hand and has some impairment in the fingers of her left hand. She sustained second- and third-degree burns on her face, chin, and mouth. She lost her eyebrows, the lower part of her nostrils, and a section of hair at the center of her scalp. She says the injury that suddenly changed her appearance and her life became the biggest opportunity for growth.

"I HAD TO ACT COURAGEOUSLY and fearlessly to get through the many challenges of recovery, rehabilitation, school reentry, and community reentry," she says. "I had to learn how to live as a survivor, not a victim." By going back to what she was doing before the accident (she'd been a junior high school teacher) and establishing her sense of purpose, she avoided feeling like a victim.

Despite the stares, comments, questions, and whispers, Kammerer Quayle forced herself to go out in public every chance she could. She forced herself to learn how to handle social situations in a friendly and open way so that even the most uncomfortable situations would be manageable. Although the unwanted attention made her sad and angry, she knew that it was better than being isolated and alone. She prayed: *God, please help me look just good enough so I can be in public without everyone looking at me.* She also sought help from a psychotherapist, whom she saw for about a year.

"Self-disclosure is a powerful tool," says Kammerer Quayle, who explained to her junior high school classes about the accident, including what her care was like and why she had to wear pressure garments. The children became a source of support for her. Following many reconstructive surgeries, she recognized that her surgeon couldn't do anything more for her and, in any case, she'd reached her limit. Her face still shows signs of discoloration and scarring and it is not as symmetrical as she'd like it to be. Although her eyebrows never grew back, her surgeon was able to restore her nostrils and improve the shape of her lips.

Through extensive research, Kammerer Quayle located a makeup artist who worked with burn survivors. She has developed a comprehensive program for image enhancement, from basic skin care and makeup application to color analysis and hairstyle, which she uses to coach survivors to be as comfortable with themselves as possible.

She also teaches survivors what she calls STEPS to social comfort and confidence: Using self-talk, what you say to yourself and believe is what you create in your life, **speak** in a friendly and enthusiastic **tone** of voice; make **eye** contact; remember your **posture** — head raised and shoulders back; and **smile**.

By nature, humans are curious animals. Most people don't stare to be rude; they stare because they're curious. "It is a reality of life that looking different draws attention," Kammerer Quayle explains. The key to dealing with staring is to rethink what it means. If several people are staring at you, you begin to internalize their action and feel self-conscious, which leads to anger, sadness, or shame. Why give strangers that kind of power? Standing up straight, looking the person in the eye, smiling — even with your eyes or by your tone of voice — and saying, "Hi, how are you?" leads to an interruption of their behavior, she says. People see you as a person and not as an object.

How you look is one thing, she says, but how you present yourself is another. "It's all about attitude! And that's what you have one hundred percent control over," she says. Kammerer Quayle admits that you cannot change the public; you can only change your attitude. "Because some person acts badly toward you does not make you a bad person; their cruelty speaks more about them than you." Come from a place of love, warmth, grace, and poise when responding to others, she advises.

Kammerer Quayle stopped allowing herself to be concerned about what she thought others thought of her. "Brains work like cassette tapes," she says. "If we have 50,000 thoughts a day, many might not be positive and some might be negative, keeping us down. If you don't like what's in your brain, change it. Start a new tape for yourself. If you can change your brain, you can change your life."

ONE YEAR AFTER GWEN had walked out of the Ohio BVR, a representative from the bureau contacted her to find out how she could help her go to college. Gwen told her she couldn't afford to go to school, but the woman persisted.

"I'd like to be a paralegal, but I can't afford it," Gwen said, explaining that she wasn't in a position to take out any loans.

"Did I ask you about loans?" the woman said. "Look, we can help you."

The woman told Gwen that she was eligible for grants; if she maintained a C average, the bureau would pay for her education. At first Gwen was incredulous, but a minute later she was walking on air. She knew she wanted to attend a small college. Even though her appearance was much improved, she knew being out in public and around other students was going to be a challenge. She applied to Myers University to get her bachelor's degree in paralegal studies.

For four years Gwen juggled her classes and surgeries, most of which she scheduled for the summer, when she had more time off. One semester, she took her classes from home because of a complex surgery. Sometimes, she'd study at the Case Western Reserve University law library until midnight. Still, the experience was making Gwen stronger. She did well in school and began feeling more confident. Her only trouble came from one man: a law professor.

In all her classes, Gwen sat in the front row so that she would be sure she was seeing and hearing everything the instructor was imparting to the students. Her law professor took exception to seeing Gwen up close.

"Why do you have to sit up front?" he asked her one day.

"I can pay attention better," said Gwen.

"You can't do that from the back?"

Gwen, trying to control her rage, asked whether he wanted her to move, to which he replied, "Yes."

After that semester was over, Gwen's professor asked her not to sign up for any more of his classes. "His were the first ones I signed up for," she laughs.

Eventually, their relationship went from ice-cold to tepid. Gwen was the only person in his class, up to that time, to get an A on an exam. The professor told Lexis, who accompanied Gwen to class one day, that her mother was a very intelligent woman. Gwen was only too happy to shine a spotlight on his ignorance for making an assumption based on her appearance. "I proved him wrong," she says, smiling.

After four years, Gwen graduated with a respectable 3.28 grade point average. Although she looked forward to a career that she'd worked hard to earn, her marriage was failing, and she and Al separated. Then she found out that she was pregnant.

EVER SINCE SHE WAS a girl, Gwen has had premonitions through dreams. The dreams always foretold a tragedy. Twice she dreamed she and her husband were in a fire. And before Gwen and Al were married, she'd asked him whether he would still love her if she didn't look the same anymore. He said, "Yes, I love you for who you are." She'd then asked him whether he would take care of her if she couldn't use her hands. "Of course," he told her.

"It's the funniest thing," says Al. "All the things she asked me about happened."

"It was almost like it had to be proven," adds Gwen.

THAT GWEN WAS UNABLE to use her hands after the fire was the only thing that prevented her from killing herself. Her sadness and anger were overwhelming and no one, it seemed, could help her. She had to figure things out on her own. Then one day, she was able to express the feeling she'd had for so long: "I'm angry at God!" She realized that if she felt angry at God, He must already know it anyway, so she might as well shout it.

"That was the first time I felt good, just saying that," she says. Then she discovered that it was too risky not to be honest about her feelings. "Give your feelings their own person; otherwise they'll take you over. That's dangerous and that's deadly. Respect them as though they're another person. It's okay to have your feelings fluctuate. Everyone is allowed to feel what they want. Let them feel," she says. "Let them feel."

After her experiences with therapy, she knew that if she could pick her sorrowful self up to leave the session, she could pick herself up anywhere. By helping herself, "no one can tell me my session is over," she says, "'cause my feelings aren't over." Gwen learned that it was okay to cry and to feel hopeless and sad, but she allows herself a safe environment in which to have those feelings. When she allows her sadness room and safety, it passes.

"If you feel like crying, cry," she says. "If you're tired of crying, move on until the next time, with the understanding that there will probably be a next time, and it's okay."

She learned that the bad feelings aren't going to disappear, though. Grief can last a lifetime. She counseled an old friend recently on this very thing, making sure to tell her that through the whole grieving process, you have to keep moving forward because if you sit too long, you won't get anywhere. "I made it to the other side," says Gwen. "Now I can reach through and pull someone else to the other side."

SOON AFTER GWEN'S SECOND daughter, Diamond, was born, she accepted a job as a customer service representative at Progressive Insurance, where she still works. Two years later, she and Al got back together, and seven years ago, they had a son, Aldurrant.

Trauma changes people — sometimes for the better, sometimes for the worse. But it always changes them. For Al and Gwen, it seems to have made them more resilient. "If I could change it, I would, but in another way, I wouldn't," says Al of the experience. Although it was painful in so many ways, the experience has improved his and Gwen's relationship. "I never thought I'd leave my wife. I loved her for her. Our relationship is so much better now. It happened nineteen years ago, and we've been married twenty-two years. I'm more used to us being this way than before the fire."

At the time of the fire, Gwen was only 22 years old. Now 42, she tries to remember how she looked then. She wonders how she would look now, how her face would age, if she hadn't been injured. What would she have looked like at 50, 65, 80? When Gwen was a child, she had the same face as her daughter Diamond. The resemblance is striking. Gwen looks into her daughter's young face and sees herself when she was that age, and she hopes she'll be able to witness how she would have looked as Diamond gets older, starting when Diamond turns 22. That's the point forward, says Gwen.

WHEN CLEVELAND CLINIC ANNOUNCED approval for a face transplant in 2004, Gwen inquired immediately. "I think it's a blessing," she says. But because her injuries aren't severe enough — her face is scarred, but her functional limitations essentially involve her hands — she doesn't qualify. "I have certain limitations, but others may have more severe injuries and loss of function."

At the time, critics of the procedure argued that a face transplant was too experimental, that the doctors involved in face transplant are trying to play God, and that people should be happy with the face God gave them.

"This is not what God gave me," says Gwen, who is passionate about the potential for the procedure. Even though some are put off by the thought of looking like someone else, Gwen says that concept doesn't bother her. When she inquired about the face transplant, she had to complete a psychological questionnaire. One question was, How would you feel looking like someone else? "It's a misconception," says Gwen. "I look like someone else now."

To the critics who accuse doctors of moving forward with face transplants just for fame or say that they're playing God, she asks, "Did you ever stop to think they're listening to God? Many days I prayed for it," she says. "Many days." Even though Gwen will not directly benefit from a face transplant, she feels that God has heard her prayers and the prayers of others who feel the way she does. To those who can't fathom the procedure because being facially disfigured isn't life-threatening, she asks, "Who are they to determine that either? I was suicidal for a year and a half! That's life-threatening! Things seemed so hopeless. Finally, here's something that's a ray of hope."

What concerns Gwen the least are people like her, who look different but are out in public, working, shopping, living. They are the people who have learned how to cope with the open-mouthed stares and the associated paranoia, the feeling that people are always pointing their fingers, whispering. It's the people with facial differences who are in hiding who weigh on her mind. They are the people who don't dare step into the daylight because they fear the reactions of others. They cannot bear to face a world that can be so unkind. Like the Phantom of the Opera and Beauty's beast, they've committed themselves to an unnatural life, living one level below the rest of civilization.

"If you're injured or your appearance is so different, you automatically stand out and people don't know how to react. People treat you like you have the plague. They run," says Gwen. "If society didn't treat people so bad, this issue may not have come up."

Says Al, "What really bothers me is how people are cruel to her. In the early years, I'd say, 'Take a picture!' Now I just keep walking. As you get older, you get wiser. People are just ignorant." And to those people, Al has words of caution: "You better be careful because it could happen to you. Your life can change in a matter of seconds," he says.

Despite the stares and rude remarks and double takes, Gwen doesn't want people to pretend her facial difference doesn't exist. "I know for a fact there's something different about me, so acknowledge that fact and move on. Don't say there's absolutely nothing wrong. I'm seeing it every day in the mirror." Her family and friends provide balance and a sense of normalcy because when they look at Gwen, they don't see the scars as scars. The scars are just a part of her, like her effusive personality, her love of laughter, her eyes full of hope, and her renewed love of life. "They genuinely and truly see me for me."

CHAPTER 14

give and take

In order to be a realist you must believe in miracles.

—David Ben-Gurion

IN FALL 2004, Dr. Maria Siemionow received approval from the Cleveland Clinic's Institutional Review Board to proceed with a full-face transplant. Suddenly, the whole world was talking. After a year, talk had died down, but then a team of French physicians performed the world's first partial face transplant and conversation erupted again.

Isabelle Dinoire, the 38-year-old recipient of the partial face transplant, had been badly disfigured by a dog attack just seven months earlier. According to Jean-Michel Dubernard, one of the lead doctors, the injuries to Dinoire's nose, lips, and chin were "extremely difficult, if not impossible to repair with classic surgery." The woman had difficulty speaking and eating. A partial face plus bone marrow to help prevent rejection were donated by the family of a woman who was brain-dead.

After the procedure, the French team was widely criticized for acting hastily in not preparing Dinoire psychologically for the transplant. Rumors circulated that she had attempted suicide by overdosing on pills prior to being mauled by the dog. What's more, Dr. Dubernard was on the team that had performed the world's first hand-forearm transplant; critics contended that he was itching to perform the world's first partial face transplant.

Despite the rumors and speculation (as well as the patient's smoking habit, which nearly compromised acceptance of the transplant early on), as of this writing, Dinoire is reported to have regained sensation in her face.

At the end of 2008, Dr. Siemionow and a team of Cleveland Clinic surgeons performed the first near-total face transplant in the United States. Roughly 80 percent of an anonymous female donor's face was transplanted onto the anonymous recipient.

Face transplant appears to be possible.

FOLLOWING THE ANNOUNCEMENT that Cleveland Clinic approved the protocol to perform the world's first full face transplant, the "gross factor" was significant. There was concern that some people would have a face transplant just to improve their average looks. This seems highly unlikely for many reasons — not the least of which is that one doesn't imagine Angelina Jolie or anyone like her giving up her face anytime soon, and the sale of body parts on eBay is prohibited. Another concern was that face transplants might be used by criminals trying to change their identities. But all this speculation is unfounded for two reasons: First, getting a face transplant won't be like ordering car parts. Even if face transplants were to become standard of care, not every doctor would have the skill to perform one. Second, criminals easily can get a nose job, liposuction, eyebrow lift, and countless other cosmetic procedures already if they want to change their appearances.

Forty years ago, controversy surrounded heart transplant, too, when Dr. Christiaan Barnard performed the world's first in December 1967. People had strong reactions to heart transplant because it introduced new ethical issues, such as conflict of interest and the definition of death. People questioned whether they would be viewed by their physicians as patients or potential organ donors. How could they be sure their physician had their best interests in mind, especially if another of their doctor's patients sorely needed a heart to survive? Where was the doctor's allegiance? People also were squeamish about transplanting a heart because of its symbolism, with its history of being connected to emotion and feeling, much as a face is connected to identity.

Most people who object to face transplant stand by their argument that having a severely disfigured face is not life-threatening, but this is not totally correct. Some people who are severely disfigured don't even leave their homes because they are so despondent. Some are suicidal, and some have killed themselves. The real question is this: Is quality of life just as important as life? Is concern with anything less than loss of life frivolous? This debate, which often is sparked with respect to euthanasia, is nothing new, but face transplant does give it a fresh forum.

Other objections are based on the grounds that our faces are too closely related to identity. We communicate through our faces; four of our five senses are on or near our faces; and we are recognized first and foremost by our faces. But changing a face — replacing tissue, rebuilding a nose, reconstructing lips — doesn't change our history, our values and experiences, or our ability to experience emotions, much as a new quilt doesn't negate the years of passion, joy, and pain that occur in the bed of a long-married couple. Our selves live deep inside us, in an ethereal space called the soul; changing one's face doesn't change who that person is.

Some people also are afraid that the face transplant recipient will look just like the donor. Cadaveric and computer-modeling studies show that, because the transferred tissue will drape over the recipient's underlying bone and musculature, the tissue will take on a hybrid look that more closely resembles the recipient than the donor. Once transferred, the recipient's new face will bear just a trace of the donor's face.

The most compelling argument against face transplantation involves the risk factors. As with any new procedure, it's difficult to anticipate or calculate all the risks, which has caused some to question the validity of the informed consent process. We do know that the long-term risks of immunosuppressive therapy are real, and they include kidney failure, diabetes, and the development of various cancers.

Since the partial face transplant performed in France and the near-total face transplant performed in the United States, the public's perception of the procedure appears to have become more positive. Dr. Siemionow, director of Plastic Surgery Research at Cleveland Clinic, thinks the reason for this shift is that people can see that a face transplant is feasible and that a person can return to a more normal life. "So it's not anymore ridiculous," she says.

Born and educated in Poland, Dr. Siemionow trained in Europe and in the United States; she has spent the last two decades researching transplantation and microsurgery, publishing dozens of papers in professional journals. Microsurgery, which is precision surgery performed using specialized instruments and a microscope, has been around for nearly 30 years, but the application to the face using donor tissue is a newer concept. By performing mock face transplants in the laboratory and on cadavers, Dr. Siemionow demonstrated that the delicate procedure of transplanting a face was possible.

But is it really necessary? Traditional repair of large injuries to the face and scalp have involved skin grafts and an assortment of flap techniques, all used with varying degrees of success from a medical standpoint, and less success from an aesthetic perspective. Skin grafts are stiff and leave an uneven, mismatched look that more often resembles a hastily fashioned patchwork quilt than a face. Tissue flaps also leave a mismatched look. For extensive facial injuries, conventional tissue flaps simply aren't large enough. And, in the case of burn survivors with extensive facial injuries, enough usable tissue is often unavailable nearby. To patch someone together using multiple flaps requires several surgeries, including one to re-create a nose, if necessary.

Surgeons have had success in using expanded tissue, along with its own blood supply, from a patient's back for a "face transplant," but tissue taken from a person's back isn't the same as facial tissue. Skin on the eyelids, for example, is the thinnest, at about 0.5 millimeters (or

0.02 inches). Most of the skin on the rest of the body is between 1 and 2 millimeters (0.04 to 0.08 inches) thick. The bottom line is that tissue taken from any other part of the human body doesn't have the same topography as facial skin.

Of tissue transferred to the face from the back, for example, Dr. Siemionow explains, "It's not pliable, it's too thick and covers fifty percent of the full facial defect." In the March 2006 issue of *Plastic and Reconstructive Surgery*, she published a paper on this topic. To repair a full facial defect, a piece of skin must be large enough to accommodate all the curves and contours of the face. Remember, the face is three-dimensional; if facial skin is ironed flat, its large size would be surprising. Without the scalp, a piece of tissue required to cover an entire face would measure about a foot by a foot, explains Dr. Siemionow. "That's a large piece of skin, if you think about it." If a scalp were needed, the amount of donor tissue required would nearly double.

Artificial skin is not a practical substitute, says Dr. Siemionow, adding that it lacks flexibility and the ability to provide sensation and function: "So far, nothing artificial works as well as human tissue."

Dr. Siemionow is adamant when she talks about the need for face transplant. She wants people to understand that the procedure is not about vanity. A face transplant is designed to restore the appearance of someone who is severely disfigured, but it also will help restore function. In the case of burn survivors, for instance, their damaged skin prevents them from sweating; they may not have eyelashes or eyelids, both of which help protect the eye; and they may have an open nasal cavity (covering it with a prosthesis may be too painful), which is a magnet for bacteria. For a person with serious functional issues, the desire for a face transplant goes far beyond improving physical appearance.

SKIN PEELS AWAY FROM the body surprisingly well. A face and scalp can be removed in such a way that all the features remain completely intact, including ears, eyebrows, hair, eyelids, nose, mustache, lips, and even wrinkles. The peeled face very much resembles a rubber Halloween mask, complete with holes for the eyes to see and the nostrils to breathe. Ghoulish, perhaps, but remarkable.

A face transplant or, more accurately, a composite tissue allograft transplantation, which refers to transplants of organs made up of multiple tissue types, is done in two stages. The first stage involves removing the skin, nerves, blood vessels, and other soft tissues, such as fat and cartilage, from the donor. Tissue must be harvested from the donor within six hours of death for it to be usable. In the case of the near-total face transplant performed at Cleveland Clinic, this stage of the surgery took about nine hours. The second stage involves removing the recipient's damaged facial tissue by making an incision from the hairline to the chin. Surgeons then must connect the recipient's blood vessels to the vessels in the tissue graft, and next use painstaking microsurgery techniques to connect arteries, veins, and nerves. In the Cleveland Clinic example, the second stage of the surgery to transplant the donor tissue lasted nearly 12 hours.

A successful face transplant will offer recipients a chance to be ordinary, to blend in more easily with society, to look like everyone else — to look mediocre, perhaps. For them, it would mean not being the center of attention, knowing that eyes weren't following them as they picked out peaches at the grocery store or pumped gas into their cars. The ability to turn heads would be a thing of the past. It's what Hollywood stars hope for and fear at the same time.

If the transplant fails, with the new tissue dying and turning necrotic, the only option is to reconstruct the face using tissue taken from other parts of the recipient's body, such as the back. That's why it's so important that the candidate for face transplant have available, usable tissue someplace else.

The biggest risk involves the need for lifelong immunosuppressive drugs and the associated risk of kidney damage and many types of cancers, including squamous cell carcinoma, which, ironically, often shows up on the face. All transplant patients need the drugs to prevent their bodies from rejecting the new organ. Although a few people have successfully been weaned from immunosuppressive drugs, it seems unlikely that this would be possible for a face transplant patient. Skin produces the strongest immune response of all organs, because its job is to protect the entire body from foreign invasion.

The need for immunosuppressive drugs is an enormous problem for all transplant patients, but it is an even larger issue with face transplant, because a facial deformity in and of itself is not immediately life-threatening, at least in the same way a failing heart is. When one's life is on the line, it's easier to accept the risk of potential future harm in exchange for life, and for some people with severe facial deformities, the risk may outweigh the benefit. Dr. Siemionow and researchers around the world are working to find ways to reduce the need for immunosuppressive drugs in transplant patients. She has had success in preliminary laboratory studies and hopes to bring the research to human trials soon in cases involving solid organ transplants, such as the transplants of the kidney and liver.

Asked whether she ever gets tired of talking about face transplant, she smiles quickly and shrugs but immediately seizes the opportunity to deliver her message: "It's important to keep up the conversation, even ad nauseam, educating people and telling them what it is not," she explains. "Like advertising cereal, even though this is a medical procedure, you have to get the message out. You don't hear anyone criticizing people for enlarging their lips or enhancing body parts, but to help people look normal, they criticize. This is not vanity or *Face/Off*," she says, referring to the 1997 movie starring John Travolta and Nicolas Cage. "It's no problem to make you beautiful, but a problem to make you look normal."

Dr. Siemionow has a clinical practice devoted to treating people with diabetic neuropathy, nerve compression, and traumatic injuries in the hands and feet. When she is not in the laboratory or seeing patients, she relaxes by taking photographs. People are her favorite subject. It doesn't matter what they look like; she's simply drawn to their faces.

BEFORE THE CLEVELAND CLINIC'S Institutional Review Board approved the full-face transplant, the 13-member panel considered every angle, every ethical concern, and every question. The board, which typically reviews and approves applications for clinical trials involving human subjects within a few weeks, took nearly a year to consider and approve the face transplant trial.

A clinical trial is just that: a trial, an experiment. Before researchers carry out clinical trials on human subjects, they must apply and get approval from a hospital's institutional review board. The IRBs are composed of medical and nonmedical people, including one member of the community. Just as with courtroom juries, the goal is to have a fair and balanced representation of people who must make extremely important decisions.

The biggest challenge to the IRB members was that the face transplant is unknown territory. Making sure the study participant understands the risks and benefits is one of the board's overarching goals. The method by which this is accomplished is through the consent form. A clinical trial consent form outlines all the known risks and benefits involved in the experiment and is purposefully written in easy-to-understand language. Particularly in complex studies like the face transplant, it's crucial that the study participant understands the consent form.

Dr. Katrina Bramstedt, a bioethicist at Cleveland Clinic, was involved early in the review process, making recommendations to improve the consent form and the psychosocial assessment. "Obviously, at the time, there hadn't even been a partial face transplant done. There was no baseline to work with as to how you would assess a potential research subject," she says. "My approach was to use the burn literature as a baseline, reading extensively about emotional, psychological, and psychiatric body image issues with people with severe facial disfigurement, and go from there." This information, as well as that gained from her review of the literature regarding hand transplantation, laid the groundwork for her bioethics approach to face transplantation.

For the face transplant study, Dr. Bramstedt's concern was to create a robust consent form. She says, "There are a couple of things we look for in bioethics regarding consent forms. One is to be sure they don't hyperinflate the benefits or underestimate the risk or somehow give the impression that the topic at hand is routine medicine or the standard of care. It's not. It's research."

To that end, she makes sure that a person who participates in a clinical trial is not called a patient but rather a research subject, recipient, adult participant, or research participant. "While this may sound callous, it's simply done so that those involved in the study — including the research participant — aren't led to believe that the study is standard of care, which is something a person gets or is supposed to get when that person is a patient," she explains.

Regarding the psychosocial risks, Dr. Bramstedt paid careful attention to how the recipient might feel about his or her face, knowing the facial tissue was from someone else. Could the recipient handle it emotionally? Even though the end result would be some hybrid look (the recipient would look neither like the donor nor himself or herself), the face still would be new, donated from someone else. Reviewing literature from hand transplants, she discovered cases in which the recipients didn't even want to look at the transplanted hand. If the recipient has difficulty accepting the transplant, he or she runs the risk of losing it through neglect or perhaps even suffering some sort of mental breakdown. "You have to be able to accept it and take care of it," she says.

What the recipient thinks about a face, the concept of a face, and why it's important also were crucial factors to Dr. Bramstedt as she considered the psychosocial aspects of the study. She wants to know what would motivate a person to seek this tremendously invasive and completely experimental procedure.

IN FALL 2005, Dr. Siemionow began conducting extensive interviews with face transplant candidates. The criteria to qualify are strict, because she considers the procedure a measure of last resort. First, the candidate must be an adult. No child would be considered because of the lifelong need for immunosuppressive therapy and its associated risk of cancers. Cancer survivors are not candidates, for the same reason. Second, the candidate must be severely disfigured; the defect must be recent. Third, the candidate must not have had much prior reconstruction; and, fourth, he or she must have enough available tissue elsewhere on the body, in the event the transplant fails. This last criterion would eliminate people who have been burned over a large part of their body.

From a psychosocial perspective, the candidate must be stable enough to cope with receiving someone else's facial tissue. Some transplant recipients develop an unhealthy bond with the donor or the donor's family.

Notoriety also is an issue. Although everything possible will be done to protect the identity of the recipient, more than likely that information will get leaked and the recipient will be thrust into the international spotlight — a far cry from the ordinary, anonymous life the person hopes to gain from having the procedure in the first place.

Having a reasonable expectation of the result is another issue. "One important thing to understand is expectations," says Dr. Bramstedt. "Do they want to look like a movie star, or do they want a basic, general improvement, one that's more socially accepted in grocery stores and in hiring practices?" The recipient also needs to understand that he or she could wind up looking worse, she adds. There is no guarantee that the procedure will be a "visual" success.

The decision to go ahead with the surgery must be made thoughtfully by the candidate. The candidate's social supports — family and friends — will be carefully considered to ensure that no one is forcing a decision. "It's so important that participation in a research study, particularly one of this magnitude, be completely voluntary and the decision made without coercion," Dr. Bramstedt says.

Finding an appropriate face transplant candidate is one thing, but finding a suitable donor is quite another. An appropriate donor must match in terms of age, sex, and skin color. Because the donor must be deceased, the donor's family must make the decision to donate facial tissue, and the considerations are quite different from those involving an internal organ. An internal organ, hidden deep inside the body, feels more like a necessary component of the entire "machine" while one is alive. Losing it after death doesn't seem so harsh. But facial tissue is so closely connected to identity and so visible that the thought of disfiguring a loved one may be too much for a family. (Family members must be willing to have a closed-casket service.) Finally, even though the recipient won't look like the donor after surgery, family members may still harbor a fear of seeing their "loved one" strolling down the street someday.

FROM THE PERSPECTIVE OF organ donation, facial tissue falls under the category of soft tissue, so technically it is included in soft-tissue donation. Before you tear up your organ donation card because you fear inadvertently donating your face, know that there is a rigorous consent process involved in being a face transplant donor. Facial transplant is so novel, it is not included in the standard donation agreement made effective by filling out an organ donation card.

Most people who are amenable to donating organs will not feel squeamish about donating facial tissue; they understand the value of giving another person a chance at life. People who are unsure about organ donation might consider what happens to the body after death within a month, within a year, within five years. The gift of life — even if it's quality of life — cannot be underestimated. We are expendable, often in life and certainly in death.

EVEN AMONG PEOPLE WITH facial differences, there is some debate about face transplants, but the dialogue has been played out mostly from a personal perspective. Either they personally would consider a face transplant or not.

Christine Piff, founder of Let's Face It, an international organization for people with facial differences based in England, wasn't always an advocate for face transplants. When she first heard about face transplants, she says she was horrified. The idea of taking tissue from a deceased person and transplanting it to a person with a disfigured face was nearly beyond belief.

But in her 22 years of working with thousands of people with facial differences, she's seen the devastation and despair that result from being shunned by society. Face transplants may be an answer.

"Especially for young people," she says, "who shut themselves away totally. They don't live, they exist. To me, they would benefit."

Piff understands the pain of having to face others when you look different. When she was 36, she lost her left eye, half her palate, and her upper jaw to cancer. After her surgery, she recalled a nurse telling her, "Christine, you still have got your eye." She wrote about the experience later, adding, "I smiled a big smile, and my teeth fell onto my chin."

Piff believes that more than half of people with facial differences hide themselves away, which is why there's such a low awareness about facial differences. If the controversy over face transplant has done nothing else, it at least has elevated awareness and given those who are badly disfigured a measure of hope.

"I don't know what the impact of a face transplant will be, but I know that the experience of having an altered face takes a lot of time to accept. People who wear a facial prosthesis, like I do, understand," says Piff, referring not only to the initial trauma, but to the ongoing refinements to the prosthesis to make sure it's "aging" along with its wearer. "I go through the same change with that prosthesis. I have to accept it. And if I don't accept it, there's trauma. I don't feel safe. I'm altered.

"The psychological drama for the patient is going to be a big one," she continues. "I think there will be a lot of counseling — for the rest of their life, probably."

That a face transplant recipient needs to take lifelong immuno-suppressive drugs isn't a factor for Piff. Although she understands the risks, she accepts that the drugs are necessary — just as they're necessary for recipients of other organ transplants. She reasons that she'd rather have five years of quality life, being accepted by society, than a longer life of being shunned.

"It's a very personal thing," she says. "Unless you've been involved with someone with facial disfigurement, it's easy to be judgmental."

People who might have been face transplant candidates and reject the idea do so for their own personal reasons. Perhaps they've grown accustomed to their faces and have accepted themselves. Some don't feel the risks are worth the possible benefits or are unwilling to undergo one more surgery.

Critics say something is just not right about having someone else's face. If face transplant isn't an option, though, shouldn't we consider our behavior and attitude toward people who look different from the rest of us?

Imagine putting on a mask of a face very different from your own and very different from what's "normal." Then try going about your daily life — going to the mall, eating at a restaurant, grocery shopping, going to work, or interviewing for a job. Make a point of walking past a group of teenagers on the street, hailing a cab, or asking someone for a date. Wear the mask day after day, pretending that you can't take it off, so there's no end in sight. It's hard to imagine experiencing the world through someone else's eyes. We can only say what we might do.

That people with facial differences can't have happy and fulfilling lives simply isn't true. The resilience of the human spirit is amazing. So many people who have suffered loss go on to be successful and give back to others. Many people with facial differences have found acceptance, made peace, and discovered grace, but there are those who haven't been that lucky. We should not pass judgment on what might be right for someone else. Not when we haven't experienced the world from behind their eyes and seen the expressions of the faces looking back at them.

※

RESOURCES

BIRTH DEFECTS

Albinism/Hypopigmentation

National Organization for Albinism
and Hypopigmentation (NOAH)
PO Box 959
East Hampstead, NH 03826-0959
(800) 473-2310
webmaster@albinism.org
www.albinism.org

Apert Syndrome

Apert Web Page
Don & Cathie Sears
PO Box 2571
Columbia, SC 29202
(803) 732-2372
catndon@apert.org
www.apert.org

Cleft Lip/Palate

American Cleft Palate Craniofacial
Association
1504 East Franklin St., Ste. 102
Chapel Hill, NC 27514-2884
(800) 24-CLEFT
24-hour hotline for parents:
(919) 933-9044
info@acpa-cpf.org
www.acpa-cpf.org

Ameriface
(formerly AboutFace USA)
Cleft Advocate
PO Box 751112
Las Vegas, NV 89136
(702) 769-9264
24-hour toll-free hotline:
(888) 486-1209
info@ameriface.org or
debbie@cleftadvocate.org
www.ameriface.org and
www.cleftadvocate.com

Crouzon Syndrome

Crouzon Support Network
PO Box 1272
Edmonds, WA 98020
(425) 672-1697
crouzons-owner@yahoogroups.com
www.crouzon.org

Freeman-Sheldon Syndrome

Freeman-Sheldon Parent
Support Group
Joyce Dolcourt
509 E Northmont Way
Salt Lake City, UT 84103-3324
(801) 364-7060
info@fspsg.org

www.fspsg.org

Goldenhar Syndrome
Support Network
Ameriface
PO Box 751112
Las Vegas, NV 89136
(702) 769-9264
24-hour toll-free hotline:
 (888) 486-1209
info@ameriface.org
www.goldenharsyndrome.org

Moebius Syndrome
Moebius Syndrome Foundation
PO Box 147
Pilot Grove, MO 65276
(660) 834-3406
vicki@moebiussyndrome.com
www.moebiussyndrome.com

Nager and Miller Syndromes
Foundation for Nager and Miller
 Syndromes
13210 SE 342nd St.
Auburn, WA 98092
(800) 507-FNMS (3667)
International: 001-253-333-1483
ddfmns@aol.com
www.nagerormillersynd.com

Neurofibromatosis
Children's Tumor Foundation
95 Pine St., 16th Floor
New York, NY 10005
(212) 344-6633 or (800) 323-7938
info@ctf.org
www.ctf.org

Neurofibromatosis, Inc.
PO Box 66884
Chicago, IL 60666
(630) 627-1115 or (800) 942-6825
www.nfinc.org

Parry Romberg Syndrome
Parry Romberg Foundation
526 14th St.
Windsor, CO 80550
info@parryrombergfoundation.org
www.parryrombergfoundation.org

Romberg's Connection
Chicago, IL
rombergs@hotmail.com
www.geocities.com/HotSprings/1018

Pierre Robin Syndrome
Pierre Robin Network
3604 Biscayne
Quincy, IL 62305
info@pierrerobin.org
www.pierrerobin.org

Proteus Syndrome
Proteus Syndrome Foundation
4915 Dry Stone Dr.
Colorado Springs, CO 80918
www.proteus-syndrome.org

Stickler Syndrome
Stickler Involved People
15 Angelina
Augusta, KS 67010
(316) 259-5194
sip@sticklers.org
www.sticklers.org

Stickler Syndrome Support Group
PO Box 371
Walton on Thames
KT12 2YS
01932 267635
info@stickler.org.uk
www.stickler.org.uk

Treacher Collins Syndrome

Treacher Collins Connection
PO Box 120416
Boston, MA 02112
(704) 545-1921
tom@tccconnection.org or
    judy@tccconnection.org
www.tcconnection.org

Vascular Birthmarks

Hemangioma Hope
8400 Rohl Road
North East, PA 16428
(814) 898-1054
cdouganHH@aol.com
www.members.tripod.com/
    ~Michelle_G/HHopeN.html

Sturge-Weber Foundation
PO Box 418
Mount Freedom, NJ 07970
(800) 627-5482
swf@sturge-weber.com
www.sturge-weber.com

Vascular Birthmark Foundation
PO Box 106
Latham, NY 12110
(877) 823-4646
www.birthmark.org

Velo-Cardio-Facial Syndrome

Velo-Cardio-Facial Syndrome
    Educational Foundation
PO Box 874
Milltown, NJ 08850
(732) 238-8803 or (866) VCFSEF5
info@vcfsef.org
www.vcfsef.org

Von Hippel-Lindau Syndrome

VHL Family Alliance
2001 Beacon St., Ste. 208
Boston, MA 02135-7787
(617) 277-5667 or (800) 767-4845
info@vhl.org
www.vhl.org

BURNS AND TRAUMA

Brain/Head Injury

Brain Injury Association of America
1608 Spring Hill Road, Ste. 110
Vienna, VA 22182
(703) 761-0750 or (800) 444-6443
www.biausa.org

Burns

Phoenix Society for Burn Survivors,
    Inc.
1835 R W Berends Dr. SW
Grand Rapids, MI 49519-4955
(616) 458-2773 or
    (800) 888-BURN (2876)
info@phoenix-society.org
www.phoenix-society.org

CANCERS

Acoustic Neuroma Association
Lois White, Executive Director
600 Peachtree Pkwy., Ste. 108
Cumming, GA 30041-6899
(770) 205-8211 or (877) 200-8211
info@anausa.org
www.anausa.org

Adenoid Cystic Carcinoma
    Organization International
San Diego, CA 92175-5482
www.orgsites.com/ca/acco

American Brain Tumor Association
2720 River Road
Des Plaines, IL 60018
(800) 886-2282 Patient Line
(847) 827-9910
info@abta.org
www.abta.org

Basal Cell Nevus Syndrome
BCCNS Life Support Network
PO Box 321
Burton, OH 44021
(440) 834-0011 or (866) 834-1895
info@bccns.org
www.bccns.org

Candlelighters Childhood Cancer
   Foundation
PO Box 498
Kensington, MD 20895-0498
(301) 962-3520 or
   (800) 366-CCCF (2223)
staff@candlelighters.org
www.candlelighters.org

Children's Cancer Association
433 NW 4th Avenue, Ste. 100
Portland, OR 97209
(503) 244-3141
office@e-cca.org
www.ChildrensCancerAssociation.
   org

National Brain Tumor Society
East Coast Office
124 Watertown St., Ste. 2D
Watertown, MA 02472
(617) 924-9997 or (800) 770-8287

West Coast Office
22 Battery St., Ste. 612
San Francisco, CA 94111-5520
(415) 834-9970 or (800) 770-8287
info@braintumor.org
www.braintumor.org

National Cancer Institute
NCI Public Inquiries Office,
   Ste. 3036A
6116 Executive Blvd., MSC8322
Bethesda, MD 20892-8322
(800) 4-CANCER
www.cancer.gov

National Coalition for Cancer
   Survivorship (NCCS)
Ellen Sovall, Executive Director
1010 Wayne Ave., Ste. 770
Silver Spring, MD 20910
(301) 650-9127
(877) 622-7937 Publications
info@canceradvocacy.org
www.canceradvocacy.org

Oral Cancer Foundation
3419 Via Lido, #205
Newport Beach, CA 92663
(949) 646-8000
info@oralcancerfoundation.org
www.oralcancerfoundation.org

Support for People with Oral
   and Head and Neck Cancer
   (SPOHNC)
PO Box 53
Locust Valley, NY 11560-0053
(800) 377-0928 or (516) 759-5333
info@spohnc.org
www.spohnc.org

SYSTEMIC AND SKIN

Foundation for Ichthyosis and
   Related Skin Types (F.I.R.S.T.)
1364 Welsh Road G2
North Wales, PA 19454
(215) 619-0670
info@scalyskin.org
www.scalyskin.org

National Alopecia Areata Foundation
14 Mitchell Blvd.
San Rafael, CA 94903
(415) 472-3780
info@naaf.org
www.naaf.org

National Vitiligo Foundation
PO Box 23226
Cincinnati, OH 45223
(513) 541-3903
info@nvfi.org
www.nvfi.org

Scleroderma Foundation
300 Rosewood Drive, Ste. 105
Danvers, MA 01923
(978) 463-5843 or
   (800) 722-HOPE (4673)
scleroderma.org

Sjogren's Syndrome Foundation
6707 Democracy Blvd, Ste 325
Bethesda, MD 20817
(301) 530-4420 or (800) 475-6473
www.sjogrens.org

Wegener's Granulomatosis
   Association International
PO Box 28660
Kansas City, MO 64188-8660
(816) 436-8211 or (800) 277-9474
vf@vasculitisfoundation.org
www.wgassociation.org

FACIAL PAIN
(including Trigeminal Neuralgia)

The Facial Pain Association
925 NW 56th Terrace, Ste. C
Gainesville, FL 32605
(352) 331-7009 or (800) 923-3608
patientinfo@tna-support.org
www.endthepain.org

CRANIOFACIAL ORGANIZATIONS

AboutFace
123 Edward St., Ste. 1003
Toronto ON
Canada M5G 1E2
(416) 597-2229
(800) 665-3223
info@aboutfaceinternational.org
www.aboutfaceinternational.org

American Anaplastology Association
9213 Mintwood St.
Silver Spring, MD 20901
(301) 495-1590 or (877) 495-1590
info@anaplastology.org
www.anaplastology.org

Ameriface
   (formerly AboutFace USA)
PO Box 751112
Las Vegas, NV 89136
(702) 769-9264
24-hour toll-free hotline:
   (888) 486-1209
info@ameriface.org
www.ameriface.org

Children's Craniofacial Association
13140 Coit Road
Ste. 517
Dallas, TX 75240
(214) 570-9099 or (800) 535-3643
contactCCA@ccakids.com
www.ccakids.com

Craniofacial Foundation of America
975 E Third St., Box 269
Chattanooga, TN 37403
(423) 778-9192 or (800) 418-3223
terri.farmer@erlanger.org
www.craniofacialcenter.com

FACES: The National Craniofacial
   Association
P. O. Box 11082
Chattanooga, TN 37401
(423) 266-1632 or (800) 332-2373
faces@faces-cranio.org
www.faces-cranio.org

Forward Face: Helping Children
   with Facial Differences
317 East 34th St., Ste. 901A
New York, NY 10016
(212) 684-5860 or (800) 393-FACE
info@forwardface.org
www.forwardface.org

Foundation for Faces of Children
258 Harvard St., #367
Brookline, MA 02446-2904
(617) 355-8299
www.facesofchildren.org

Let's Face It
University of Michigan
School of Dentistry /
   Dentistry Library
1011 N. University
Ann Arbor, MI 48109-1078
faceit@umich.edu
www.dent.umich.edu/faceit

Let's Face It UK
72 Victoria Avenue
Westgate On Sea
Kent CT8 8BH
01843 833724
chrisletsfaceit@aol.com
www.lets-face-it.org.uk

National Foundation for Facial
   Reconstruction
317 East 34th St., Room 901
New York, NY 10016
(212) 263-6656
www.nffr.org

OTHER

National Institute on Deafness and
   Other Communication Disorders
National Institutes of Health
31 Center Drive, MSC 2320
Bethesda, MD 20892-2320
nidcdinfo@nidcd.nih.gov
www.nidcd.nih.gov

National Organization on
   Disability (NOD)
910 Sixteenth St. NW, Ste. 600
Washington, DC 20006
(202) 293-5960
ability@nod.org
www.nod.org

Washington State Fathers Network
Kindering Center
16120 N.E. Eighth St.
Bellevue, WA 98008-3937
(425) 653-4286
greg.schell@kindering.org
www.fathersnetwork.org

For a complete list of resources, including books, videos, and product information,
e-mail or visit Let's Face It at faceit@umich.edu or www.dent.umich.edu/faceit.

CHAPTER REFERENCES

INTRODUCTION

Miranda Hitti. "CDC Lists Top 6 Types of Birth Defects." WebMD. Available at http://www.webmd.com/content/article/116/112412.htm. Accessed June 4, 2006.

Erving Goffman. *Stigma: Notes on the Management of Spoiled Identity*. New York: Simon & Schuster, Inc., 1963.

Malcolm Gladwell. *Blink: The Power of Thinking Without Thinking*. New York: Little, Brown and Company, 2005.

Elizabeth Austin. "Marks of Mystery." *Psychology Today*. Available at http://www.psychologytoday.com/articles/pto-19990701-000032.html. Accessed November 24, 2004.

Mike Grundmann, Producer. *The Perfect Flaw*. Videocassette. 2002. 26 min.

Yale Medical Group. "Facial Trauma May Cause Significant Social and Behavioral Problems." May 2005. Available at http://www.yalemedicalgroup.org/news/ymg_persing.html. Accessed June 4, 2006.

CHAPTER 1

Benjamin Barankin and Gordon E. Searles. "Nevoid Basal Cell Carcinoma." Emedicine. 2004. Available at http://www.emedicine.com/ped/topic1592.htm. Accessed May 2, 2005.

American College of Mohs Micrographic Surgery and Cutaneous Oncology. "About the Mohs College." Available at http://www.mohscollege.org/AboutMC.html. Accessed June 4, 2006.

Guinness World Records. "Most Operations Endured." Available at http://www.guinnessworldrecords.com/content_pages/record.asp?recordid=48461. Accessed August 15, 2005.

CHAPTER 2

Donald H. Enlow and Mark G. Hans. *Essentials of Facial Growth.* Philadelphia: W.B. Saunders Company, 1996.

Henry Gray. Gray's Anatomy. 15th ed. New York: Barnes & Noble Books, 1995.

G.J. Tortora and S.R. Grabowski. *Principles of Anatomy & Physiology.* 10th ed. Hoboken: John Wiley & Sons, Inc. 2003.

Arthur I. Miller. "A Thing of Beauty." New Scientist. February 4, 2006:50–52.

"The Mathematical Formula for the Perfect Face!" June 11, 2004. Available at http://www.cojoweb.com/phi.html. Accessed June 5, 2006.

BBC News. "China Crowns Miss Plastic Surgery." December 18, 2004. Available at http://news.bbc.co.uk. Accessed September 14, 2005.

Celeste Biever. "For a New Personality, Click Here." *New Scientist.* February 25, 2006:30.

Michael Howell and Peter Ford. *The True History of The Elephant Man.* New York: Schocken Books, 1980.

Robert J. Gorlin. *Facial Folklore.* Mead Johnson Symposium on Perinatal and Developmental Medicine. 22(1983):43–47.

John B. Mulliken and Anthony E. Young. *Vascular Birthmarks: Hemangiomas and Malformations.* Philadelphia: W.B. Saunders Company, 1988:3–9.

W.C. Shaw. "Folklore Surrounding Facial Deformity and the Origins of Facial Prejudice." *The British Journal of Plastic Surgery.* 34(1981):237–246.

DataFace. "Facial Expression: A Primary Communication System." Available at http://face-and-emotion.com/dataface/expression/expression.jsp. Accessed February 13, 2006.

CHAPTER 3

Louise Ashby. *Magic of the Mask.* London: John Blake Publishing Ltd., 2001.

CHAPTER 4

Canada & World War One — the First Contingent. "Repairing Maimed Faces." Available at http://groups.msn.com/CanadaWorldWarOnetheFirstContingent/repairingmaimedfaces.msnw. Accessed November 15, 2004.

M.H. Kaufman, J. McTavish, and R. Mitchell. "The Gunner with the Silver Mask: Observations on the management of severe maxillofacial lesions over the last 160 years." *Journal of the Royal College of Surgeons Edinburgh.* 42(December 1997):367–375.

Health Superstore. "Plastic Surgery History." Available at http://www.healthsuperstore.com/ articles/plastic-surgery-history.aspx. Accessed December 9, 2004.

Christian Medical College, Dodd Memorial Library. "Susruta—Surgeon of Old India." Available at http://dodd.cmcvellore.ac.in/hom/06%20-%20Susruta.html. Accessed June 4, 2006.

Michael Ciaschini and Steven L. Bernard. "History of Plastic Surgery." eMedicine. Available at http://www.emedicine.com/plastic/topic 433.htm. Accessed November 18, 2004.

Thomas V. DiBacco. "Altered Images: Plastic Surgery's Earliest Cases Date to Ancient Egypt, India." *The Washington Post*, December 13, 1994. Available at http://www.hindunet.org/alt_hindu/1994_2/msg00097.html. Accessed November 18, 2004.

Elizabeth K. Hale. "The History of Flaps." *Journal of Drugs in Dermatology.* 1(December 2002):293.

Project Façade. "Gen. Yeo Piece1: Setting the Scene." December 20, 2005. Available at http://www.projectfacade.com/index.php?/news/comments/gnr_yeo_piece_1_setting_the_scene. Accessed October 23, 2006.

Craig Williams. "Harold Gillies: Aesthetic Reconstructor." Nzedge.com. June 2002. Available at http://www.nzedge.com/heroes/gillies.html. Accessed June 4, 2006.

Andrew Bamji. The Gillies Archives at Queen Mary's Hospital, Sidcup. Available at http://website.lineone.net/~andrewbamji/archives.htm. Accessed June 4, 2006.

Francis A. Countway Library of Medicine. "Varaztad H. Kazanjian (1879–1974)." Available at http://www.countway.harvard.edu/rarebooks/exhibits/plastic_surgery/page_2.html. Accessed November 26, 2004.

Lce Snowden. Corp. Fred. Letter to Varaztad Kazanjian. September 24, 1918.

Kevin W. Lobay. "Varaztad Kazanjian: Life and Times." The Proceedings of the 12th Annual History of Medicine Days." Faculty of Medicine, University of Calgary. Ed. W.A. Whitelaw. March 21–22, 2003. Available at http://www.hom.ucalgary.ca/Dayspapers2003.pdf. Accessed June 4, 2006.

Harvard Medical Alumni Bulletin. Winter 1962:8–9.

Medical News Magazine. Interview with V.H. Kazanjian. Vol. 23, No. 5, May 1979.

Wikipedia. "Plastic Surgery." Available at http://en.wikipedia.org/wiki/Cosmetic_Surgery. Accessed October 23, 2006.

Project Façade. "Anna Coleman Ladd and Francis Derwent Wood." January 1, 2005. Available at http://www.projectfacade.com/index.php?/about/comments/anna_coleman_ladd. Accessed October 23, 2006.

CHAPTER 5

Berlin Center for Facial Prostheses/Anaplastology. "From 'a Gold Nose' to the Modern Facial Prosthesis." Available at http://www.gesichtsepithetik.de/eng/history.html. Accessed November 10, 2004.

David Jansen and Moises Salama. "Facial Alloplastic Implants, Mandibular Angle." eMedicine. Available at http://www.emedicine.com/plastic/topic52.htm. Accessed November 15, 2004.

American Society of Ocularists. "Frequently Asked Questions." Available at http://www.ocularist.org/faq.html. Accessed June 28, 2005.

Frank McDowell. *The Source Book of Plastic Surgery*. Baltimore: The Williams & Wilkins Company, 1977.

CHAPTER 6

Patricia Bacon Smith. "Tessier Clefts." Available at http://www.cleftline.org/som/0301/Tessier%20Info.pdf. Accessed June 4, 2006.

Robert Naseef. *Special Children, Challenged Parents: The Struggles and Rewards of Raising a Child with a Disability*. Baltimore: Brookes Publishing Co., 2001. http://www.alternativechoices.com.

Frances Cooke Macgregor. "Facial Disfigurement: Problems and Management of Social Interaction and Implications for Mental Health." *Aesthetic Plastic Surgery*. 14(1990):249–257.

Erving Goffman. *Behavior in Public Places*. New York: The Free Press, 1963.

Let's Face It USA. *Resources for People with Facial Differences*. 2005/2006.

U.S. Equal Employment Opportunity Commission. "Facts About the Americans with Disabilities Act." Available at http://www.eeoc.gov/facts/fs-ada.html. Accessed October 19, 2005.

CHAPTER 7

David Roche. "My Face Does Not Belong to Me." Available at http://www.davidroche.com/face.htm. Accessed November 26, 2004.

Frances Cooke Macgregor. "Facial Disfigurement: Problems and Management of Social Interaction and Implications for Mental Health." *Aesthetic Plastic Surgery*. 14(1990):249–257.

CHAPTER 8

Jeffrey A. Fearon. "Pfeiffer Syndrome." *FACES Today*. 13(Spring 2005):5.

CHAPTER 9

Sara Rosenfeld-Johnson. Innovative Therapists International. http://www.talktools. net. Rick Guidotti. Positive Exposure. http://www.rickguidotti.com.

CHAPTER 10

cleftAdvocate. http://www.cleftadvocate.org. AboutFace USA. http://www.about faceusa.org.

CHAPTER 11

Fathers Network. http://www.fathersnetwork.org.

Kathleen A. Kapp-Simon. "Psychological Care of Children with Cleft Lip and Palate in the Family." In *Cleft Lip and Palate: From Origin to Treatment.* Diego F. Wyszynski, ed., Oxford University Press, 2002.

Patricia Bacon Smith. "Tessier Clefts." Available at http://www.cleftline.org/som/0301/ Tessier%20Info.pdf. Accessed June 4, 2006.

Cleft Palate Foundation. "About Cleft Lip & Palate." Available at http://www.cleftline. org/aboutclp. Accessed March 3, 2006.

Wide Smiles. "Tessier Facial Clefts." Available at http://www.widesmiles.org/syndrome /tessier. Accessed March 3, 2006.

CHAPTER 12

Tim Bonfield. "Doctor Traveling Long Way to Repair Deformed Faces." The Enquirer. July 1, 2005. Available at http://news.enquirer.com/apps/pbcs.dll/article ?AID=/20050711/ NEWS01/507110337/1056. Accessed August 19, 2005.

University of Cincinnati Medical Center. "Extreme Makeover May Lead to Discovery of Gene Mutation." Medical Center Findings. October 2005. Available at http:// medcenter.uc.edu/pr/findings/makover.cfm. Accessed September 30, 2005.

Patricia Bacon Smith. "Tessier Clefts." Available at http://www.cleftline.org/ som/0301/Tessier%20Info.pdf. Accessed June 4, 2006.

Larry Thompson. "Human Gene Therapy: Harsh Lessons, High Hopes." *FDA Consumer.* September-October 2000. Available at http://www.fda.gov/fdac/ features/2000/500_gene.html. Accessed June 5, 2006.

P.H. Warnke, I.N.G. Springer, and J. Wiltfang, et al. "Growth and Transplantation of a Custom Vascularized Bone Graft in a Man." Lancet. 364(2004):766–70.

Catherine Arnst. "The Dynamic Duo of Tissue Engineering." *BusinessWeek.* 1998. Available at http://www.businessweek.com/1998/30/b3588008.htm. Accessed January 24, 2005.

Mary Carmichael. "Organs Under Construction." *Newsweek.* Summer 2005:46–48.

Nancy Fliesler. "The Graft that Keeps on Giving." *Dream*. Children's Hospital Boston. Spring 2005:21–24.

CHAPTER 14

CNN.com. "Woman 'Has First Face Transplant.'" November 30, 2005. Available at http://www.cnn.com/2005/HEALTH/11/30/france.face. Accessed November 30, 2005.

MSNBC. "Face Transplant Patient Makes an Appearance." February 6, 2006. Available at http://www.msnbc.msn.com/id/11198533. Accessed February 7, 2006.

David J. Rothman. *Strangers at the Bedside: A history of how law and bioethics transformed medical decision making*. New York: Basic Books, Inc. 1991.

Celeste Biever. "Man's Face Rebuilt with Single Skin Graft." NewScientist.com. October 13, 2004. Available at http://www.newscientist.com/article.ns?id=dn6520. Accessed February 24, 2006.

G.J. Tortora and S.R. Grabowski. *Principles of Anatomy & Physiology*. 10th ed. Hoboken: John Wiley & Sons, Inc., 2003.

Maria Siemionow, Sakir Unal, Galip Agaoglu, and Alper Sari. "A Cadaver Study in Preparation for Facial Allograft Transplantation in Humans: Part I. What are alternative sources for total facial defect coverage?" *Plastic and Reconstructive Surgery*. 117(March 2006):864–872.

Peter Gorner. "Surgery's Next Step: Face Transplants." *Chicago Tribune*. June 12, 2005.

ABOUT THE AUTHOR

LAURA GREENWALD is senior manager, creative services/editorial, at Cleveland Clinic in Cleveland, Ohio. In that capacity, she has overall responsibility for the editorial content of consumer, physician, and corporate marketing communications. She is founder of the Healthcare Communicators Network, a group of communication professionals from top medical centers across the United States. She earned her bachelor's degree in marketing from Notre Dame College of Ohio and lives in Chardon with her husband, Scott.

More information about *Eye of the Beholder* is available at http://heroeswiththousandfaces.blogspot.com. A portion of the author's proceeds benefits programs to support people with facial differences.